Building the Client Bond S

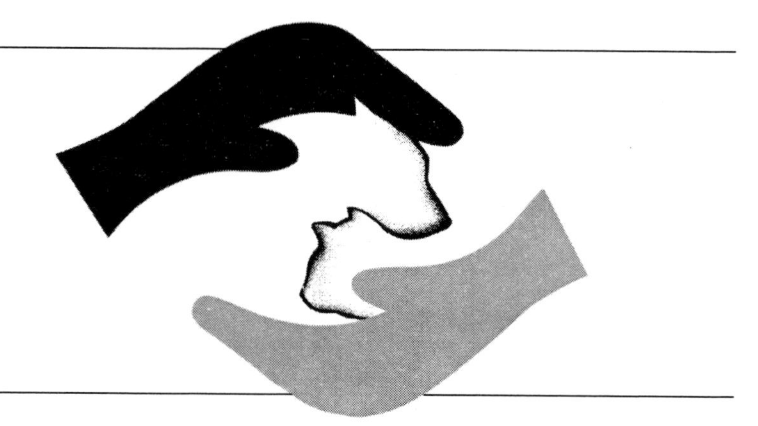

Connecting with Clients

Practical Communication Techniques for 15 Common Situations

Laurel Lagoni, M.S.
Co-founder and former Co-director

and

Dana Durrance, M.A.
Assistant Director

Changes: The Support for People and Pets Program
Colorado State University Veterinary Teaching Hospital

AAHA Press

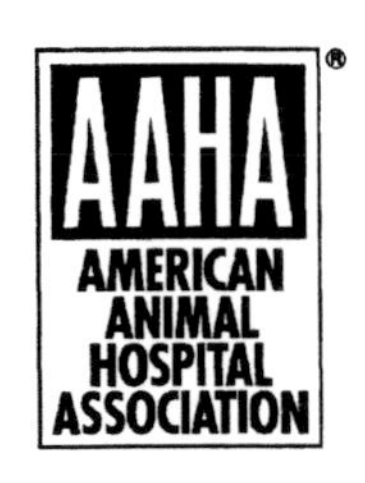

First published in the USA by AAHA press, a division of the
American Animal Hospital Association
12575 West Bayaud Avenue
Lakewood, Colorado 80228

ISBN 0-941451-67-4

This book was designed and produced by
AAHA Press

Many thanks to the AAHA Press Editoral Advisory Board:
Dr. Laurel Collins, ABVP
Dr. Richard Goebel
Dr. Charles Hickey
Dr. Clayton McKinnon
Dr. Richard Nelson, ABVP
Dr. Hal Taylor

Design and Typography
Sheryl Tongue

Cover Design and Illustration
Dave Bonick

Dedications

This series is dedicated to my friends and colleagues at both Colorado State University (CSU) and the American Animal Hospital Association (AAHA). Their joint efforts and financial support saved Changes: The Support for People and Pets Program in 1989 when it was in danger of being terminated due to a lack of funds. Thank you all for believing that creating positive relationships with clients is worthy of our collective emotional, intellectual, financial, and professional investments.

I would also like to dedicate this particular guide to my own 15-year-old dog Toby who died this year. —L.L.

I dedicate this book to my husband, Steve, and to my daughter, Erin, whom I was pregnant with while writing chapters for this book. To Steve, thank you for your constant support of my career and for introducing the Changes program to me when you were a veterinary student at Colorado State University. Thank you for sharing your experiences as a practicing veterinarian; I learn from you every day and marvel at the job that you do. To Erin, thank you for keeping me company while writing and for giving me good healthy kicks along the way!

I would also like to dedicate this book to the companion animals that I have loved: Gretchen, Schroeder, Millie, LaVerne, and Mindy. I miss you all so much. Finally, I dedicate this book to my two other "daughters," Roxanne and Pfeiffer. Thank you for your canine silliness, your wisdom, and for all the love that you bring to our home. With you, I know that the human-animal bond is one of the most beautiful forces in this world. —D.D.

Acknowledgements

No book comes about in isolation. For this series to come to fruition, my co-author Dana Durrance wrote outstanding versions of most of the communication strategies even while she was eight months pregnant and about to begin her maternity leave. Dana, the current Changes Program assistant director, deserves much of the credit for this book's readability and quality. Thank you, Dana. I literally could not have delivered this book on time without you. You have accomplished two wonderful deliveries this year!

At the American Animal Hospital Association, four women in particular played important roles. Debby Morehead, AAHA's former acquisitions editor, had the original idea and enthusiasm. While writing this series has been rewarding, the greatest personal rewards have come from getting to know Debby as a friend and colleague. Also deserving of credit is Judy Mazarin, AAHA's former publications coordinator. Judy initiated this project, thus allowing me to continue to have a voice in veterinary medicine. Two other professionals came later to this project and lent their considerable editing, marketing, and management skills to it. Dana McCullah and Toni Smith deserve much of the credit for this series being innovative, practical, and attractive to users. I respect their professionalism and high standards and look forward to future projects with them.

Gratitude is extended to the veterinarians, veterinary technicians, AAHA staff members, and other colleagues who contributed to the revision and production phases of this project. Their insights, comments, and guidance were invaluable and the content and scope of this project is more realistic and useable because of them.

Finally, my personal gratitude is extended to W. B. Saunders Company and to Carolyn Butler, M.S., and Suzanne Hetts, Ph.D., my co-authors on *The Human-Animal Bond and Grief.* Without their clinical innovations and professional collaboration, many of the concepts in these guides would not exist. —L.L.

I would like to thank Laurel Lagoni for her support and invitation to share in writing this book. Laurel, you have been a pioneer in recognizing the importance of the human-animal bond in veterinary medicine. Without you, there would not be a Changes Program at Colorado State University. You are an inspiration to me and to the thousands of pet owners, veterinarians, students, and others whom you have helped through your remarkable talents in counseling, teaching, and writing.

To Carolyn Butler, the Director of the Changes Program, I owe you a debt of gratitude that is nearly impossible to express. You have created opportunities for me that have literally changed my life. You have taught me, guided me, and been the kind of mentor that most people dream about. Thank you for sharing your incredible skills and allowing me to contribute to a program like Changes. Most of all, I want to thank you for your friendship and for the collaboration that we enjoy.

I would also like to acknowledge the staff at AAHA for their assistance in making this book as well as the many people involved in the revision and editing.

I would like to express my gratitude and appreciation to the faculty, staff, students, clients, and patients of the teaching hospital at Colorado State University. It is through working with you that I have learned so much about the human-animal bond and have witnessed amazing experiences inspired by the love and beauty of that bond. —D.D.

Authors' Notes

We directed this text to veterinarians even though we realize many other veterinary professionals (technicians, receptionists, office managers) may read and benefit from these communication techniques. In fact, these techniques are most effective when all members of a veterinary team consistently use them together.

The communication techniques described in this book are designed to be effective with the majority of your average veterinary clients. It's important to remember, though, that there are often individual differences that must be taken into consideration when it comes to effective communication. Age, gender, culture, religious orientation, and a host of other factors can influence how clients respond to your attempts to connect with them. If you feel the communication technique you are using is not effective, it may be that another technique would be more appropriate based on your client's unique needs.

Table of Contents

Foreword ix

Preface xi

Client Communication Concepts
What You Need to Know

Who is This Book For? 2

How to Use This Book, ... 3

As a Preparatory Guide 3

As a Professional Growth or Teaching Tool 3

The Human-Animal Bond 5

The Human-Animal Bond and Communication 6

Communication Basics 7

Non-Verbal Communication 8

Verbal Communication 8

Communication Techniques 9

Verbal Techniques 10

Non-Verbal Techniques 12

The Limits of Client Communication 13

Communication Strategies
How to Connect with Clients in 15 Common Situations

Situation 1: How Your Clinic Environment Conveys that You Care 16

Situation 2: Establishing Trust and Rapport 19

Situation 3: Clients' Needs, Problems, and Concerns 22

Situation 4: Listening 25

Situation 5: Body Language 28

Situation 6: When You Must Say "No" 32

Situation 7: Indecisive Clients 35

Situation 8: Resolving Differences and Misunderstandings with Clients 38

Situation 9: When You Need to Apologize 41

Situation 10: Humor 44

Situation 11: Complaining or Demanding Clients 47

Situation 12: Fearful and Anxious Clients 50

Situation 13: Angry Clients 53

Situation 14: Clients with Financial Constraints 56

Situation 15: Grieving Clients 60

The Telephone and Clients Relations 62

Caught in the Act 63

Communication Feedback Form 64

References 65

Resources 67

Glossary 69

Meet the Authors 71

Foreword

A Lesson in Relationships

By Merry Crimi, DVM

In The AAHA Report we discovered that at least 70 percent of pet owners describe their pets as children. Since that awakening, many have tossed the term around, sometimes almost as a distant and impersonal reference to a "category" of clients. As veterinarians, we see many pet owners every day that we recognize in this group. Some make us smile. Some make us uncomfortable. Some we pass off on associates because they take too much time. The AAHA Report served as a wake-up call for all companion animal practitioners. At least 70 percent of pet owners expect us to act more like pediatricians in the relationships we have with them. At least 70 percent expect that we will recognize, honor, and respect the bond that ties them to the animal whose health they entrust to us. An episode I experienced today may seem unusual to some, but typifies many of the experiences that touch our lives in practice every day.

This afternoon I got a call from Patty, a long-time client who owns a 15-year-old poodle named Bunky. Patty and Bunky have been frequent fixtures in my exam room for Bunky's entire life. I have been saddened on visits during the past two years as I've watched Bunky become crippled with back and joint disease. Recent visits have brought the inevitable discussions about aging changes, pain, and the decision process surrounding euthanasia.

Making a bit of extra time for listening on each visit over the last 15 years helped me understand a lot about Patty and Bunky's relationship that was critical in our communication today. I learned through trust and time about Patty's loss of her only baby a week before its expected birth date many years ago. I knew about a painful divorce from the man who would never let her keep those baby's ashes or have more children. I knew about her father, who died recently. A man she still calls "Daddy."

Patty is very much a "pets-as-children" client. Those who have no time for their clients might have labeled her flaky. They wouldn't understand why she always insisted on carrying her 40-pound dog. Or why she had an irrational fear of bad news, even when Bunky was in for routine vaccinations. They wouldn't know that today, when Patty had to make a decision to euthanize Bunky, she was severing a tie to the one thing that had helped her survive all of life's worst imaginable traumas. Today she had to let go of the only warm thing she could ever hold.

Sadly, there are a lot of Pattys out in the world today. Some are brave enough to tell their stories to those who listen. Many are not or never get the chance. If we as veterinarians assume that at least 70 percent of pet owners see their pets as children, we will hopefully push ourselves to give the time, understanding, and respect to every pet owner we see. If we listen a lot and care a lot we can have the good fortune of knowing many whose lives are touched and sometimes saved by the incredible ties between animal and man.

These special pets come in many shapes, sizes, and ages, as do the clients who depend on them. This afternoon it was a woman and a poodle. This morning it was a gerbil with his nine-year-old boy. Tomorrow it might be a diabetic cat with a single, elderly man or a cockatoo clutched by a young girl.

Veterinary medicine is about relationships. It's about the animals who need us for good health and the people whose lives these animals live to enrich. It's about rewards far greater than the paychecks we bring home. Rewards far greater than the interesting science and technology that we master.

If we try to categorize the pet owners we see in order to figure out what level of care they'll want or focus only on minimizing exam room time to squeeze more clients in our day and increase the net profit, we will never really be able to celebrate the real reasons we chose veterinary medicine as a career. The power of the human-animal bond is a mighty force. It gives each of us the privilege of connecting and serving the public on a level that few others can know. If you want to take one piece of The AAHA Report at a time to change the way you practice, I highly recommend spending a few weeks making a constructive assumption that each and every client coming into your hospital has just the connection that Patty and Bunky did. If you seek this opportunity on each client contact, you'll suddenly start enjoying the special art of veterinary medicine. The other rewards will follow.

Dr. Merry Crimi was the 1996–1997 AAHA president.

Preface

Welcome to the "human" side of veterinary medicine! This book was written to provide you with simple, basic information about how to connect and communicate more effectively with clients, thus enhancing your client relations skills. While positive client relations will make your practice more profitable in the long-run (people will feel comfortable, understood, and cared about, and therefore, return to your practice), client retention and profitability are *not* the main goals of effective communication. The main goals are to truly connect with other human beings and to make each communication interaction you're a part of clear, productive, and personally satisfying.

A series of positive communication interactions leads to deep connections or bonds between clients and veterinarians. Knowing how to build strong client bonds is the heart and soul of successful veterinary practices.

The information in this book is based primarily on the knowledge and skills gleaned through Changes: The Support for People and Pets Program at the Colorado State University Veterinary Teaching Hospital (CSU-VTH). The Changes Program was created in 1984 and today is the most comprehensive, on-site veterinary client support program in the world. When the Changes Program began, little was known about what would and would not be helpful to the pet owners who brought their beloved companion animals to the CSU-VTH. In addition, staff members were unsure about how to handle issues like client complaints, client anger, or the stress of the veterinary medical professionals with whom they worked. However, as time-tested techniques were applied to what research revealed about effective communication, certain strategies emerged as being much more useful than others. Many of those strategies are included in this book.

All pet owners who truly love their cats, dogs, horses, birds, rabbits, or any other animal deserve to be treated with respect and have important information conveyed to them with patience and clarity. It is the responsibility of all veterinarians to ensure that this happens. You can accomplish this by learning how effective communication works and incorporating basic verbal and non-verbal communication techniques into each interaction you have with clients.

The overall goal for this book is to provide you with applicable, easy-to-under-stand information about *what to say and what to do* in a variety of common client-relations situations. Rather than using a lot of theory, detailed background information, or textbook methodology, this book is filled with phrases and actions designed to give you quick and easy access to the communication strategies known to be *the most useful and effective.*

An important point to understand is that there are very few "right" or "wrong" ways to connect and communicate with clients, and the reality is that a communication strategy that works well for one person may not work as well for another. However, there *are* communication strategies that, in general, are *the most effective ones to use with the majority of pet owners and situations* you will encounter during your professional life.

Of course, there is much more to be learned about the human-animal bond, communication, stress, and helping pet owners deal with grief than you will glean from this *Building the Client Bond* series. The following information represents only the essential knowledge and skills you need. If you wish to read more about these topics, there are several recommended books listed in the Resources section on page 67.

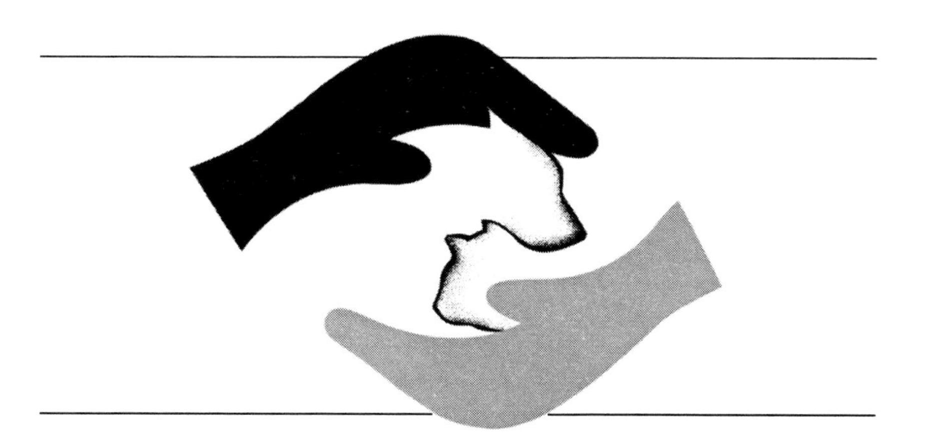

Client Communication Concepts

What You Need to Know

Who is This Book For?

This book is intended for use as both a personal reference and as a model for staff development. It is designed to help you and your co-workers get through many of the client relations situations you encounter on a day-to-day basis while on the job in veterinary medicine. It is for:

- increasing your personal knowledge about the results of effective communication
- improving your own client-relations skills
- providing your staff with the training and skills they need to incorporate effective communication techniques into their daily work
- dealing with your own communication challenges

Veterinary Technicians

- enhancing your professional growth

Office Managers

- improving client retention
- improving staff retention

Receptionists

- learning new ways to deal with difficult communication-related situations

How to Use this Book

There are two basic ways to use this book:

- *As a Preparatory Study Guide*
  This method encourages you to anticipate the issues and circumstances of your upcoming cases and to read about some of the words and techniques you might try when you're actually face-to-face with clients. This method works best when you have prior warning about the issues that may arise, like cases that involve anger or client complaints.
- *As a Professional Growth or Teaching Tool*
  This method encourages you to "process" the cases you have just been involved with by analyzing what you did well and what you might have done better. This learning process can take place on your own as you read about the situations you were involved with and the suggestions about how they could be handled. The learning process can also be used as a case study for "debriefing" during staff meetings.

  Debriefing means talking openly with your co-workers about the emotional, as well as the medical, aspects of your cases and receiving feedback and support for the communication techniques and course of action you elected to take. When you participate in a debriefing session, you present the emotional and medical elements of your case, describe what the communication challenges and emotional dilemmas were for you and the pet owner, and talk about the strategies you tried. In other words,

  a) explain what you felt went well ("This technique really worked!"),

  b) explain what you felt didn't go so well ("Mrs. James seemed to get angry with me when I suggested she might want to pay her bill ahead of time."), and

  c) ask for ideas from your colleagues regarding other ways to handle the situation ("How do the rest of you deal with suggestions that seem to offend clients?").

  If you and your co-workers enjoy a fairly high level of trust and mutual respect, it might be interesting to use your experiences with challenging client relationships as the basis of some role playing exercises. Role playing allows you to actually try out the words and strategies suggested by others.

They also allow you to play the roles of your own clients in order to gain some empathy for their points of view. Participating in role playing exercises can be intimidating, but if you feel you can trust one another to provide feedback in gentle, constructive ways, try them. Sharing experiences, both rewarding ones and embarrassing ones, is the only way to learn from your own mistakes and successes, as well as those of others. If you are secretive, defensive, or even modest about your own attempts to communicate with and help clients, little progress toward becoming more effective can be made.

Some special features are included in this guide. They are designed to help you learn to become a more effective communicator. For example, each Communication Strategy entry has an area titled "Strategies" at the end where you can record your own personal notes regarding what worked and what didn't work in each particular situation. Recording and occasionally reviewing your notes will help develop your own unique vocabulary, communication style, and customized reference guide. Write down the phrases, gestures, ideas, and methods your clients seemed to respond to in a positive way so you can be sure to repeat them next time you face that same situation.

There is also a feedback form you can use as a discussion tool during debriefing sessions and staff meetings. The best way to use this form is to make multiple copies and make it readily available for staff members to use. Be sure to also create a way that you and your co-workers can receive feedback confidentially.

Finally, there is also a list of references and resources for those of you who would like to read more about this topic, and a glossary is included for easy reference to the language of effective communication.

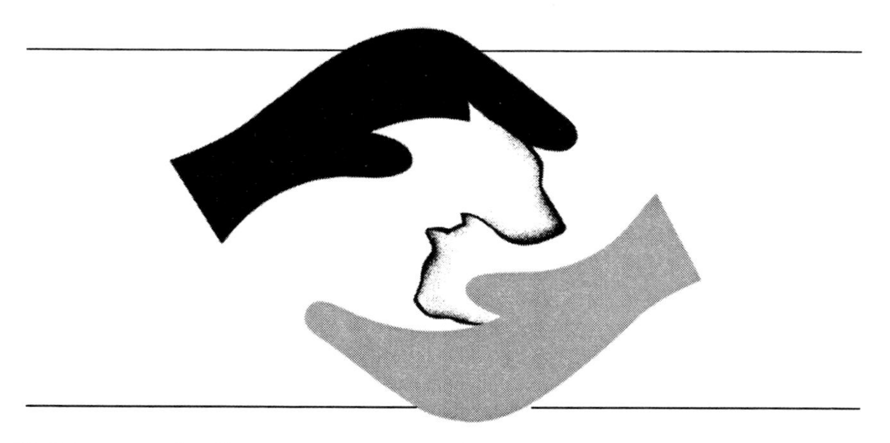

The Human-Animal Bond

Today, more people share their lives with companion animals than with children.[1] One survey tells us that 99% of dog and cat owners consider their pets to be full-fledged family members.[2] The AAHA Report reveals that at least 70% of pet owners consider their "pets as children."[3]

This deep connection with companion animals may be due to the fact that there are more single, divorced, childless, widowed, and elderly people living alone than ever before in the history of western society. In addition, we tend to move a lot in our society, often choosing to live hundreds of miles away from our close relatives and friends. Therefore, pets have become the constant presence in many of our lives and have moved into the roles traditionally reserved for other humans. These roles include confidante, mentor, child, parent, brother, sister, and best friend. Some pet owners even describe their companion animals as soulmates.

Surveys and clinical experience tell us that people often cite companionship, acceptance, emotional support, and unconditional love among companion animals' most significant and pleasing character traits.[4] There is also mounting scientific evidence that pets are good for humans, helping to maintain the physical health and psychological well-being of their owners. For example, pets have been shown to reduce high stress levels by lowering human heart rate and blood pressure.[5] They have also been known to aid in the recoveries of heart attack survivors and to act as positive agents for people undergoing various types of medical, psychological, and physical therapy treatments.[6]

If you are familiar with animal lore, you know the media frequently report on companion animals who heroically save their owners' lives. The popular media also feature animals who, more quietly but just as heroically, serve on a day-to-day basis as service animals or guides, becoming their owners' eyes, ears, and even hands. These emotional and heartwarming stories have one thing in common—they are testimonials to the power of the human-animal bond.

The term "human-animal bond" has become a popular way of referring to the types of relationships and attachments people form with animals, particularly companion animals like dogs, cats, birds, horses, goats, rabbits, snakes, ferrets, and guinea pigs. The concept of bonding with an animal is more profound than it first seems. Bonding with an animal implies making a commitment; taking responsibility; and allowing the animal

> When the deep feelings pet owners have about their pets are trivialized or when client relations issues like complaints, anger, or grief are not acknowledged with sincerity and respect, many pet owners become dissatisfied, disillusioned, and even hostile.

to influence and impact your own attitudes, behaviors, decisions, and plans. Bonding also implies that you allow an emotional attachment to an animal to occur, that you allow yourself to feel genuine affection and even love for an animal, and that you recognize and respect the fact that the animal is most likely bonding to you in return. This mutually felt bond can be immensely rewarding.

On the other hand, strong bonds can cause pet owners and veterinarians to experience great distress, particularly when their relationships with companion animals are threatened by illness or injury, or when they are trivialized in some way. These situations can create client-relations nightmares unless you know how to truly connect with clients in order to calm their anxieties, comfort them during grief, and repair any breach that may have occurred in the trust and rapport between you.

The Human-Animal Bond and Communication

In human medicine, surveys show that, along with patients' wishes for respect, courtesy, honesty, and sincerity, they also want physicians to attend to their emotions and really listen to their concerns.[7] In other words, they want doctors to be competent professionals and sensitive listeners. They want to know medical professionals are committed to helping them and that they will "stick it out" with them, even when the going gets rough. In short, they want to know that their physicians care. In fact, studies examining patient satisfaction with human medicine report that caring is more valued in the doctor/patient relationship than curing.[8] It can be assumed that veterinary clients want the same from you.

According to marketing studies, veterinarians are most often compared to pediatricians.[9] Like pediatricians, veterinarians are viewed as caregivers for the most vulnerable members of families—those who can not speak or make decisions for themselves.

Pet owners also see veterinarians as authority figures. Even though they are often quite intimidated by veterinarians, they also depend on them for guidance and emotional reassurance. The veterinary medical professional's role is an influential one and this influence makes positive client relations an extremely important issue.

According to Cecilia Soares, a California veterinarian and marriage and family therapist, inadequate communication between veterinarians and clients is the leading cause of client dissatisfaction.[10] In support of her claim, Dr. David McConnell, Trust Representative for the AVMA Professional Liability Insurance Trust, reports that communication failures trigger a significant number of malpractice claims against veterinarians.[11]

When the deep feelings pet owners have about their pets are trivialized or when client-relations issues like complaints, anger, or grief are not acknowledged with sincerity and respect, many pet owners become

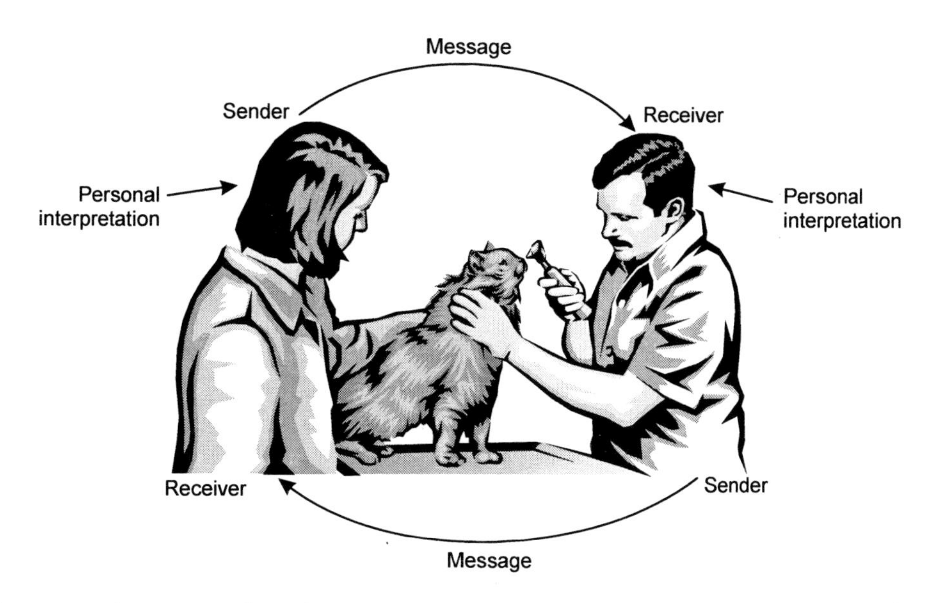

Figure 1 The interpretation steps taken during communication (Soares 1989).

dissatisfied, disillusioned, and even hostile. You can avoid many upsetting encounters with clients by becoming a skilled communicator and by learning how to build positive bonds with your clients.

Communication Basics

You might believe people are born knowing how to communicate. Yet, experts say effective communication techniques are learned[12] and that they improve with practice. Olympic swimmers are born with natural talent, but need to work hard to perfect their skills. The comparison holds true for effective communicators.

The Latin word "communis," which means "common," is the root of the word communication. Communication with another person means you try to find a common language, common experiences, and common attitudes. The goal of effective communication is to truly connect with others, finding common ground for discussion, problem-solving, creativity, and the transference of information.

Every communication process is made up of four basic elements.[13]

1) The sender—the person who speaks or conveys the message that is intended to be sent.
2) The message—usually an idea, thought, emotion, or piece of information.
3) The receiver—the listener or observer, the person for whom the message is intended.

   When these three elements work effectively, they create a feedback loop. In a feedback loop, the roles of sender and receiver alternate and information is passed back and forth successfully.

4) Interpretation

Interpretation is the fourth important element in communication.[14] Think about it. Sometimes the message that is received is not the one you intended to send.

Receivers determine the meaning and significance of the words you speak based on many other considerations, like the gestures you use, your facial expressions, and even your tone of voice. Messages are also influenced by time, the environment, and the nature of the relationship between you and the person with whom you are communicating.

Dr. Soares notes that many established veterinarians complain that new graduates are deficient in their abilities to communicate with clients.[15] Dr. Jacob Antelyes voices this same thought,

> *We were and still are so forward looking, so intent on bettering our technical skills, that we have neglected to consider the importance in our work of human relations aptitudes and communications capabilities.*
>
> *To answer the deniers and the demurrers, I only need to point to many of the help-wanted ads in the Journal. What qualities do the 'progressive' practitioners in every state seek? They want to employ veterinarians who are 'compassionate,' 'caring,' 'client-oriented,' and 'friendly,' and 'who possess communication skills.' Obviously, employers feel the need (and the lack) of these qualities in contemporary veterinary medicine.*[16] *(p. 1534.)*

Clearly, a focus on building positive client-relations and using effective communication strategies in the practice of day-to-day veterinary medicine is desirable.

Non-Verbal Communication

You may be surprised to learn that the majority of messages sent between people are conveyed non-verbally. In fact, psychologist Albert Mehrabian says only seven percent of our ideas and emotions are communicated to one another with words.[17] More specifically, Mehrabian has found that 38 percent of a message's impact comes from vocal cues (voice tone, volume, pitch, rhythm, etc.) and 55 percent from body movements (facial expressions, hand gestures, postures, etc.). That means 93 percent of our thoughts, ideas, and feelings are communicated without words.

Non-verbal communication is also *what* is said, *where* it is said, *how* it is said, *why* it is said, *when* it is said, and *who* it is said to. It is also what is *not* said. Non-verbal communication is conveyed through facial expressions, body postures, gestures, and hand movements. We are also communicating when we write, read, gesture, and listen.

The non-verbal part of communication is important because it helps people interpret or "add meaning" to what they are hearing. For example, as you work with clients, begin to notice how their body language and eye contact differ from one situation to another. Start by observing how unhappy or angry clients use closed body language and divert their eyes, while happy, confident clients use open body language and direct eye contact. Notice also how your clients' use of direct and indirect eye contact and open or closed body postures evoke the same responses from you. Remember, in a communication feedback loop, you alternate between the positions of sender and receiver. Therefore, watch your clients' eye contact and body language and be aware of your own as well!

When we communicate, we expect that peoples' words will match their facial expressions, gestures, tone of voice, and body language. If their words say one thing and their behavior says something else, it can be very confusing. Therefore, non-verbal and verbal communication must be congruent.

The term "congruent" means an "agreement of fit."[18] It means that your non-verbal and your verbal messages are compatible and that the message given verbally matches the one that is broadcast by the body.

Verbal Communication

With verbal communication, what you say is not as important as how you say it. The context in which your words are spoken has the greatest impact on the message you are trying to convey.

The effectiveness of verbal communication is affected by the words you choose; your grammar; and the tone, volume, and pitch of your voice. Effectiveness is also affected by the emphasis and inflection you place on certain words and the pacing of your overall speech. Research says that voice tone and pacing have the most influence on the meaning of spoken words.[19] For instance, if you use appropriate words to describe a situation, but speak very fast, you may be seen as rushed, nervous, insensitive, or unsure of yourself. If you speak the same words too slowly, though, you may be viewed as dull, boring, or even condescending. It's especially important for you to control your voice tone and pacing when you are working with clients who are anxious, angry, grieving, or upset because words that are spoken softly and at a slightly slower pace than normal are viewed as more soothing and comforting.

The words you use are also important. According to researchers Campbell and Helper,[19] when health care professionals use medical jargon, clients view them as more credible and their confidence in them increases. However, jargon can also alienate clients. Therefore, if technical medical terms must be used you should also explain them in plain language. For example, the word lymphosarcoma is an unknown term to the average pet owner while the word "cancer" is very familiar. Therefore, when delivering this diagnosis, you should also use the word "cancer." When you and your clients share an understanding of the meaning of words, you connect on common ground. That's when true communication begins.

Becoming an effective communicator takes practice. It takes commitment to confront problems and complaints rather than walk away from them. It also takes dedication to ongoing skill building and training. As the great educator and family therapist Virginia Satir said about communication,

> *You can read about swimming, you can watch others swim, but you don't really know what it's all about until you take the plunge yourself.*[20]

> The effectiveness of verbal communication is affected by the words you choose; your grammar; and the tone, volume, and pitch of your voice.

Communication Techniques

To communicate effectively with clients, especially when there are misunderstandings, you need to have the proper tools available to you. You wouldn't begin surgery without knowledge of anatomy and the proper instruments and equipment. Likewise, you shouldn't begin the communication process without appropriate communication techniques.

When you communicate, your goal is to be warm, clear, organized, and honest to ensure your message is sent properly for the receiver. You can present yourself this way by choosing your words carefully and by using direct eye contact, touch, and congruent facial expressions and body language.

Following are fourteen basic verbal and non-verbal communication techniques. You will find these techniques referred to over and over again in the "Communication Strategies" section. As you read the examples, think about the voice tone, facial expressions, etc., you would use in order for your message to be congruent and helpful to your client.

Verbal Techniques

Acknowledging

To acknowledge is to recognize the existence or truth of something. Acknowledging encourages people to deal openly and honestly with both the emotions that arise within them and the reality of the situation at hand. "Julie, I understand you're upset because you believe I charged you too much for Dusty's dental exam."

Normalizing

To normalize is to lend credibility to others' thoughts, feelings, and behaviors. This validates their experiences. For example, the symptoms of grief can seem quite disturbing when they are not clearly understood. It is helpful to normalize grief with statements like, "I would expect you to cry about Ruby. You two were together for ten years and were best friends. It's normal to miss her."

Giving Permission

Giving permission means encouraging clients to think, feel, and behave however they need to (within safe limits) without fear of judgment. This technique also allows clients to ask for what they want or to make requests that are important to them. For instance, if a client is anxious before her pet has surgery, she may want to wait at your clinic until surgery is completed. "I know you and Ruby are very close. If you would like to wait here until her surgery is completed, it's perfectly fine with me."

Asking Appropriate Questions

By asking questions, you gain valuable information about the circumstances surrounding your clients' needs, problems, complaints, or concerns. Failure to ask clients questions can lead to more difficulties as there are many consequences to making assumptions about your clients' needs.

The most helpful questions are open-ended, rather than closed-ended. A closed-ended question can be responded to with "yes," "no," "fine," or another one- or two-word answer. Open-ended questions elicit more detailed information and create opportunities for clients to tell you more about what they are experiencing.

Open-ended questions begin with "how" or "what" rather than with "why." "How" and "what" questions elicit thoughtful explanations. "How can I help you explain Ruby's illness to your daughter?"

"Why" questions often elicit "I don't know" answers. "Why" questions also have a tendency to put clients on the defensive, making them feel they need to explain themselves to you. One word of caution...a well-placed, open-ended question can launch a lengthy client monologue, so don't use them when you have a limited amount of time to spend with clients.

Paraphrasing

Paraphrasing is the restatement or summary of a client's communication in order to test your understanding of their comments. When you paraphrase a client's comments, it reassures the client that the intended message got through. It also provides the client with the opportunity to clarify what was meant if your understanding is inaccurate.

When paraphrasing words and emotions, it is important to paraphrase voice tone and pacing as well. If a client is speaking quickly and loudly, you should respond in a voice that nearly corresponds in volume and energy. For example, if you paraphrase anger using a slow-paced, quiet voice void of emotion, your client may feel you are being patronizing. This is likely to elicit more anger or even sarcasm from your client. While you don't want to yell or scream at a client, when paraphrasing anger, you do want to speak boldly, using a firm voice. As rapport develops and you gain some control over the situation, lowering your voice and slowing your pace may, in turn, slow down your client's side of the conversation and create an atmosphere more conducive to communication.

There are many ways to paraphrase. Easy ways to begin paraphrase statements are, "It seems like...," "It sounds like...," and "If I hear you correctly, you feel... ." A final way to use paraphrasing is to summarize the main points of a lengthy conversation in order to ensure that you've understood your client's concerns. One example of paraphrasing is,

> **Client:** I don't know how I'll ever find the money to treat Ruby's illness.
>
> **Veterinarian:** You're worried that you can't afford to help Ruby get better.

Self-Disclosure

Self-disclosure is briefly sharing a personal experience when it may be appropriate and of use to clients. Self-disclosing about your own experiences can help your clients feel more connected to you. When using self-disclosure, it is very important not to shift the focus away from your client onto yourself. An example of effective self-disclosure is, "I was unhappy with something my own physician did last month and felt I needed to discuss it with her, yet, like you, I was unsure about how to bring it up in our conversation. I didn't want to offend her or damage our relationship."

Gentle Confrontation

Gentle confrontation can be used to point out discrepancies or inconsistencies in what has been said or done. It can also be used to set limits on clients' behavior or expectations. Gentle confrontation may take the form of a question or a statement. Here are some examples of gentle confrontation:

> **Client:** You don't care at all about what happens to me or my dog!
>
> **Veterinarian:** I wonder if you really believe that. You've been bringing Ruby to me for almost four years and, together, we've helped her through many medical problems. I wonder if your harsh words today are really your anxiety about Ruby's current illness?
>
> **Client:** I know it isn't your fault that you were out of town yesterday when I needed you.
>
> **Veterinarian:** I hear a lot of anger in your voice and yet you say you're not angry.

Clients in need, or those who are upset or angry, are often demanding and obnoxious. Due to their strong emotions, they may behave in ways that they would otherwise not dream of behaving. Gentle confrontation is a necessary communication technique as it helps you set limits. With it, you can sensitively, but firmly, help clients understand your own limitations, as well as the established policies of your practice. For example, you can say something like:

> **Veterinarian:** It's obvious to me that you are disappointed that you can't stay with Nugget overnight. I know this is disturbing to you. However, I feel I have been very clear with you, from the start, regarding our policies. As I've said, we do not allow owners to spend the night in our clinic.

Gentle confrontation may also be used to narrow the content of the client's conversation. Some clients ramble on about topics unrelated to animal care, making it difficult for you to cover pertinent topics with them. Clients sometimes steer conversations off-track because they don't want to make difficult decisions or hear what you have to say. Gentle confrontation allows you to redirect conversations that have gotten off-track. You can say, for example:

> **Veterinarian:** I'd like to hear more about your son's wedding when we have more time, but right now we need to make some decisions about Ruby's treatment before I move on to my next patient.

Immediacy

Immediacy combines gentle confrontation and self-disclosure. The purpose of immediacy is to comment on the unspoken feelings or thoughts that exist within an interpersonal relationship. The use of immediacy requires you to talk openly with your clients about what you are feeling or experiencing right now. For example, you might say:

> **Veterinarian:** Sharon, I feel like something just changed between us. Did my last comment offend or hurt you in some way?

Using immediacy to comment directly on clients' thoughts, emotions, and behavior may be intimidating, so it is most effective when used within a well-established relationship. If it is used too soon or too harshly, clients may feel exposed or judged and react defensively.

Non-Verbal Techniques

Structuring the Environment

When emotions are high, people tend to get "frozen into position." They forget they can stand up if they're sitting, walk around the room if they're standing, or even leave the room altogether if they need a few minutes to be alone. This rigidity can be overcome by adapting the physical elements of your environment to better meet whatever situation is at hand.

Structuring the environment means paying attention to the various elements of your office, examination rooms, and consultation areas that can be easily moved and changed, paying attention to how chairs are arranged and how the furnishings in the room convey comfort, warmth, and understanding. The goal of structuring the environment is to "invite" your clients to communicate about their emotions instead of covering them up.

Examples of structuring the environment are placing chairs so conversations can take place face-to-face without barriers like desks or examination tables between you and your clients, or adapting examination rooms so euthanasias can be performed on the examination table, the floor, or even on a gurney rolled over near the window so the pet and pet owner can be near the outdoors.

Attending

Attending makes use of body language to convey that careful attention is being paid to the person who is talking. When your body posture is open, your eye contact is direct, and you are leaning slightly forward toward the speaker, you are demonstrating your availability and willingness to be of service.

Attending behaviors include non-judgmental facial expressions, encouraging gestures, affirmative head nods, and direct observation of what is occurring. Examples of attending behaviors include sitting down if your client sits down and squatting down to be at a child's eye level when greeting or talking to them directly.

Active Listening

There is a difference between merely hearing someone and actively listening to what they say. Active listening means listening for feelings, rather than the factual content of conversations. Active listening incorporates paraphrasing, asking questions, and attending behaviors such as eye contact and open body posture in order to encourage clients to say more. Two minor, but important, non-verbal active listening techniques are necessary silences and minimal encouragers.

Necessary Silences: When emotions are high, it is tempting to "babble" in order to fill in the silent, empty spaces; yet, remaining silent while others vent their feelings or gather their thoughts is often far more helpful.

Minimal Encouragers: Minimal encouragers are simple responses that encourage people to continue talking. The purpose of minimal encouragers is to let people know you are actively participating in the communication taking place between you. Minimal encouragers include head nods, eye blinks, and phrases like "Uh huh," "I see," and "For instance?"

Responding with Touch

Touch provides comfort, demonstrates care and concern, and often takes the place of reassuring words. Touch often has a calming affect and can help people slow their thoughts and steady themselves emotionally. There is some scientific evidence that touch affects the body physiologically, slowing heart rate and lowering blood pressure. Touch can be used to soothe a grieving client or to bring someone who is rambling back to the point.

When using touch with clients, neutral or "safe" areas to touch are the shoulders and arms. Areas of the body that are not viewed as neutral or safe include the neck, hands, torso, lower back, and legs. In general, people dislike being patted on their backs or heads. This behavior connotes a sense of superiority on your part and can be viewed as condescending. If touching or hugging clients makes you uncomfortable, a substitute technique is to touch your clients' companion animals with care. Pet owners often judge your sensitivity based on how you handle their pets.

Demonstrations

Demonstrations are a way to simplify and to "walk clients through" complicated and overwhelming medical information or procedures. Verbal descriptions generally accompany demonstrations. When used together, verbal descriptions and demonstrations give clients a step-by-step idea about what needs to be done for their companion animals.

When clients have a visual understanding of what certain treatments entail, it is often easier for them to decide whether or not those options are right for them. Videotapes are available that demonstrate the key points of several treatment protocols, and surgical procedures. Offering these videotaped demonstrations to your clients to watch, either at your clinic or at their homes, can also aid in their decision-making processes.

Written Information

Providing clients with written information is another form of non-verbal communication. Much of the medical jargon and information familiar to you is very foreign-sounding and unfamiliar to average pet owners. Therefore, it helps to write things down or to draw pictures for clients. Drawings and written materials also allow pet owners to take information home so they can describe their pets' situations accurately and in full detail to the other members of their families.

Limits of Client Communication

When you recognize the significance of the human-animal bond and become skilled at communication, you often develop a caring (and extremely loyal) clientele.

Many of your clients will grow to think of you as a friend. Once they have experienced the quality of your care, they may naturally turn to you for assistance with the other problems in their lives. For example, they may come to you with questions about a personal illness they are coping with, their child's struggle to recover from a severe injury, or the death of one of their close relatives or friends. These conversations will be emotional and it will be tempting for you to try to help them in some way.

However, you must focus your communication on the issues that arise *specific to the treatment of a companion animal*. As much as you'd like to help a client learn to face the impending death of her elderly father, *you are not trained to do so*. Your job is to acknowledge her feelings, express the compassion you feel for her dilemma, and refer her to an appropriate human service professional. As a veterinarian, your communications with clients should focus on the thoughts, feelings, behavior and problems associated with their companion animals.

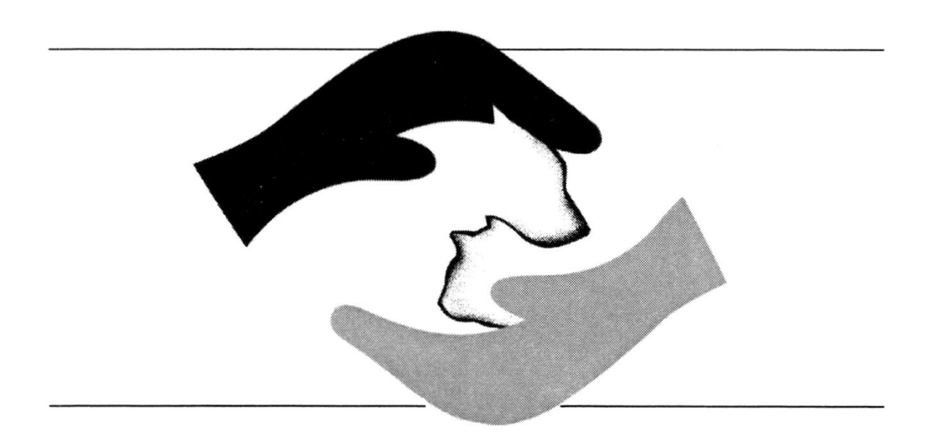

Communication Strategies

How to Connect with Clients in 15 Common Situations

Situation 1

How Your Clinic Environment Conveys that You Care

Dear Dr. Peters,

I wanted to thank you for the excellent care you gave to Sebastian during his surgery. From the very first time I brought him in to see you, I could tell that your clinic was a caring, warm place.

As a mother with two small children, I can't tell you how nice it was to have a little play area in your waiting room. My kids stayed busy and it allowed me to focus my attention on Sebastian when I knew he needed me the most. I was also impressed by the way in which you let me visit Sebastian during the three days he was hospitalized at your clinic. It was so comforting to be able to sit with him for a few minutes in one of your exam rooms. The soft pads and blankets you provided allowed me to sit right down on the floor with him and gave us some important time together that I feel was instrumental to his recovery.

I was afraid that Sebastian might have thought that I had "abandoned" him and it was so reassuring that you recognized our need to be together during this really stressful time. Your kindness and consideration clearly demonstrate your compassion and dedication to your patients as well as your clients. I am very impressed with your clinic and know that Sebastian is in the very best hands with you. Thank you again.

Sincerely,
Julie Hanson

What's Going on Here?

First impressions of your veterinary hospital or clinic can make or break a relationship with a client. Most pet owners entering a clinic for the first time make judgments about your facility on appearances first, experiences second. One of the quickest and most effective ways to instill confidence and establish trust and rapport with your clients is to have a physical environment that conveys warmth and compassion. You can easily connect with many clients just by structuring the physical space around you in aesthetically pleasing ways. If you can create an atmosphere that communicates your understanding and appreciation of the significance of the human-animal bond, you will impress many pet owners before you ever say one word.

How Can I Connect?

The goal in creating a warm and caring environment at your clinic is to structure your environment so it helps clients relax. A relaxed client is easier to communicate with, is more trusting and willing to talk, and is

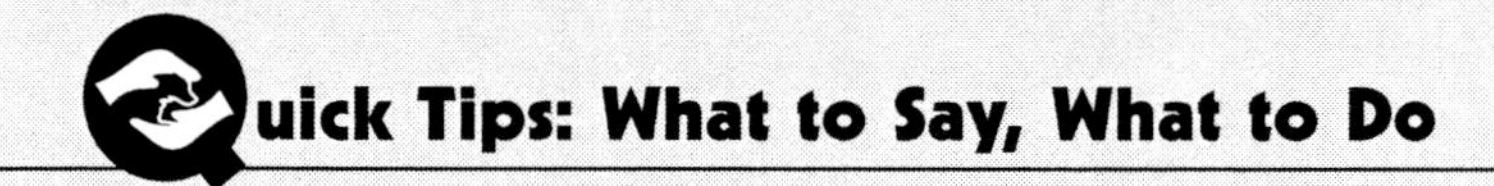

Quick Tips: What to Say, What to Do

- Keep your clinic clean and organized. This creates the perception of competence and professionalism.
- Add warmth to sterile medical environments by imposing "softer" images upon your surroundings. These might include:
  1) Outside landscaping. Flowers, trees, and grass are welcoming and friendly. They can relax people and make them feel "invited" into your facility.
  2) Softer overhead lighting in the waiting area, as well as optional lowered lighting in exam rooms for visiting times or euthanasias.
  3) A small play area for children in the waiting room with toys, books, or activities.
  4) Soft music in the waiting area. Water bowls for animals who may be thirsty.
  5) Magazines or books that promote and celebrate the human-animal bond.
  6) A small table with a supply of coffee, tea, and water for clients.
- Provide soft pads or blankets for clients and animals to sit or lie down on during visit or euthanasias in the exam rooms.
- Keep boxes of tissues in waiting areas and exam rooms.
- Provide comfortable, extra-large seating (benches) in exam rooms for you, your clients, and their families so you can sit down together to talk.
- Display pet memorials, plaques, or tributes in your waiting area. This shows you honor animals who were special to the practice and demonstrates that you understand, and take seriously, pet loss and grief.
- Install mini-blinds on exam room windows for client privacy and provide "Do Not Disturb" signs for the doors.
- If possible, provide a television monitor and videocassette player to show educational videos.

less likely to be demanding. Minor details and small comforts may seem relatively unimportant compared to the quality of your medicine, but are very important to the perceptions of your clients. The judgments and assumptions people make based on physical appearances are very powerful and lasting. If you take the time to make your environment friendly, warm, and professional, pet owners will assume that you, too, are friendly, warm, and professional.

In the competitive field of veterinary medicine, you want your practice to connect with the pet owners in your community. Your challenge is to convince pet owners that your clinic or hospital is the best place of care for their animals. The physical characteristics of your practice environment can acknowledge, normalize, give permission, self-disclose, and even "touch" clients before you utter a single word.

The physical characteristics of your practice environment can acknowledge, normalize, give permission, self-disclose, and even "touch" clients before you utter a single word.

How Will I Know if I've Been Successful?

If you have made people feel comfortable and relaxed from the very minute they walk in your door, you have gone a long way towards establishing trust and rapport and creating a positive, successful relationship with them. You might find that when clients are relaxed, your job is much easier because you don't have to put as much effort into your communication or "selling" of your practice. This is an excellent time saver for busy veterinarians like yourself. You will know that you have been successful when you have more time to direct your energies towards practicing the very best medicine that you can.

Strategies:

Situation 2

Establishing Trust and Rapport

Client: *Why can't I go back with you and hold Dugan while you take care of him? I don't want to leave him right now.*

What's Going on Here?

Clients may be wary and even suspicious of your motives for a variety of reasons. For instance, their hesitancy may be based on a previous negative experience or simply be the result of a collection of life experiences. When it comes to the health and well-being of a beloved companion animal, though, wariness may become exaggerated, especially when it comes to medical or surgical procedures that non-medical people don't understand.

> The most effective way to deal with distrustful clients is to establish trust and rapport early.

When pet owners entrust you with the care and well-being of their animals, they often perceive themselves to be powerless. This feeling of helplessness paired with a lack of control over their pet's present situation can create anxiety or fear resulting in distrust.

The most effective way to deal with distrustful clients is to establish trust and rapport early. Trust is a confidence or belief in someone's goodness and integrity. Rapport is a harmonious and useful relationship or communication. Trust and rapport are the cornerstones of any effective communication.

How Can I Connect?

Trust and rapport usually develop naturally over time, but they can be enhanced with some simple techniques. While building trust and rapport, patience is important. Some clients will automatically distrust you without any legitimate or rational reason. Try not to get defensive or to take it personally. Their lack of trust probably has little to do with you and more to do with their own experiences with the veterinary medical community in general. Some people who have also had negative experiences with professionals in human medicine will transfer some of those feelings to you because they lump you into the same category of "doctor." Some additional ways to counteract your client's distrust and develop rapport are:

- **Show interest in your clients' personal lives.**
  Chris, the last time you were in with Scooter, you were adding a new addition to your house. How is that going?

- **Compliment clients on how they care for their companion animals.**
  Scotty has lost weight since the last time I've seen him! I remember that we talked about his diet and the trouble with feeding him table scraps. You told me how hard it was for you to say `no' to his begging, but you've done an excellent job at following the recommendations. That's great.

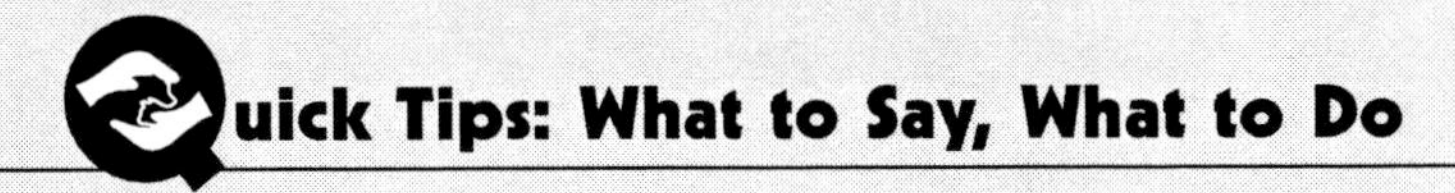

Quick Tips: What to Say, What to Do

- Self-disclose with small talk or casual conversation to make your conversation "human" and to find the common ground that you share. Some people are intimidated by professionals, especially doctors, and seeing you as an ordinary human being with the same interests and concerns as them will help clients relax.
- Normalize your clients' concerns or uneasiness:

  When I take my children to the pediatrician, I have a hard time leaving them alone. It's so hard when you love someone and are concerned.
- Touch and talk to your clients' animals. The quickest way to your client's heart is to demonstrate that you have a sincere liking for and interest in their pet.
- Communicate warmth and sincerity with your words and non-verbal behavior. Be open and approachable and use active listening, paraphrasing, direct eye contact, and open body posture. Always handle your client's animals gently and handle your client's feelings compassionately.
- Use immediacy if the client appears unusually distrustful or suspicious:

  Mrs. Atkins, I realize that we've just met and that you don't know me very well. I also realize that you are uncomfortable leaving Duggan here and seem very concerned about the care he'll receive. Can you help me understand why you feel that way? Has something happened that I should be aware of?
- Maintain your client's confidentiality. Unless you have permission to discuss a case, anything of a personal nature that your client confides in you must be kept between the two of you.
- Perform procedures in the exam room in the client's presence whenever possible.

- **Encourage clients to ask questions.**
  Many people are naturally apprehensive about medical procedures of which they have little knowledge. It is important for you to take the initiative here because many people will not tell you when they don't understand the meaning of complex medical information. Clients may even nod their heads and appear to understand because they don't want to look foolish or ignorant in front of you.

How Will I Know if I've Been Successful?

You will have to judge, on a case-by-case basis, how much effort you put forth in establishing trust and rapport with each client. When the trust and rapport is solid, your clients will be more likely to follow through on treatment recommendations, follow medical instructions, and pursue follow-up care. This is good news for your patients and you will probably find that your communication with clients flows naturally and positively. Unfortunately, there are some clients who might never feel comfortable. If you've made sincere efforts, their inability to trust you does not mean you haven't done a good job; it might simply be that they are not able or ready to place their trust in you to the extent that you deserve.

Strategies:

Situation 3

Clients' Needs, Problems, and Concerns

Lorna Murphy and her eight-year-old son Jim have a sick cat named Ida. Ida's illness can be treated, but the treatment is expensive. The clients are very attached to their pet, but don't have enough money to pay for the treatment. They are both beside themselves with grief and guilt.

Veterinary medicine is your livelihood and you must resist the urge to give your services away for free. Therefore, there seem to be only two alternatives here—euthanize Ida or donate your time and effort free of charge to her treatment.

What's Going On Here?

Most of us in the medical professions are more comfortable avoiding the feelings associated with a problem and dealing strictly with the facts. Thus, we often shut down our own emotional responses to a client's dilemma and concentrate on problem-solving. Often, we do this before we're even completely sure what the problem is.

It's important for you to realize, though, that understanding the full extent of the feelings involved with your clients' problems is just as important as gathering the complete facts of their situations. For instance, in the case above, taking a few minutes to empathize with your client's sadness and to help her explore her feelings, alternatives, and resources might greatly increase the likelihood of arriving at a solution that meets both of your needs better than either euthanasia or pro bono treatment.

How Can I Connect?

Before you attempt to meet your clients' needs or address their problems and concerns, it's helpful to evaluate your own communication skills. For example, you might ask yourself the following questions:

Is this a problem to which I am qualified to respond?

Do I know of other resources that would be more appropriate for Lorna to use?

Do I really have the time, energy, and interest it takes to follow Lorna's case through to resolution?

If you determine that finding a solution to Lorna's problem is partly your responsibility, begin to evaluate her concerns by asking her to tell you more about her feelings. You may find that, in addition to her guilt about money, Lorna feels devastated because she feels she should have noticed Ida's symptoms sooner and she is afraid that her son will blame her for the advanced state of Ida's disease. Recognition of these additional feelings gives you a clearer picture of Lorna's needs. It also tells you that both Lorna and Jim probably need some education about the probable cause of their cat's condition. They might also appreciate a referral to a human services professional who could help them deal with their guilt. Examples of resources Lorna and Jim might draw on are family and friends, other professionals such as therapists, doctors, or religious leaders, and you, as their vet-

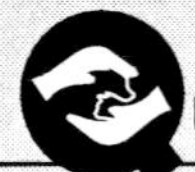

Quick Tips: What to Say, What to Do

- Acknowledge and normalize your client's feelings:

  Lorna and Jim, I can see you love Ida very much and want to find a way to help her survive this illness. Anyone who cared as much about a pet as you two do would feel sad and guilty if they thought that there was no way they could afford treatment.

- Self-disclose about your own feelings, goals, and limitations and invite the clients to work with you to find another solution:

  I don't feel right about euthanizing Ida when I can see how much she means to you, yet I can't afford to treat her for free. Dealing with the cost of treatment is the hardest part of my job, yet I know from experience that, if we take about fifteen minutes to work together, there's a good chance we can think of a solution that will work for both of us. Are you willing to work with me?

- Ask open-ended questions that will help your client explore her feelings. Try to learn more about the feelings they identify. For example, if Lorna says she feels "horrible," ask her to tell you more about that feeling.

  How is Ida's illness making you feel horrible?

- Use active listening, attending behaviors, touch, and paraphrasing to facilitate a frank discussion of your client's needs, problems, and concerns.

- Help your client generate a list of options and alternatives. Start this list by stating the range of medical options, including euthanasia, that are available to the client. You may also offer a suggestion or two regarding any financial alternatives that would be agreeable to you (payment plan, a slight reduction in fees) and any ideas you have about where she might find assistance.

  Lorna, which of your friends and family members understand how you feel about Ida and may be willing to help you?

- Structure the environment so the client can be alone in a quiet room to collect her thoughts and to sort through her options. Provide her with paper and a pen and any clinic tours, demonstrations, or written materials that may help with her decision-making process. Encourage her to call friends or family members who might be able to assist her. Gently explain that you have other patients to attend to and that you will check back with her in ten or fifteen minutes. Follow through with your promise! If the situation is not an emergency, send your client home, giving her time to explore her options further.

- Be prepared to make referrals to local support groups or to therapists who are sensitive to human-animal bond issues. The general rule about making referrals is to give clients information about how to contact resources, but let them make the actual connection themselves. The more clients do for themselves, the more control they feel over their situations.

- Maintain your client's confidentiality. Unless you have permission to discuss a case, anything of a personal nature that your client confides in you must be kept between the two of you.

- Support your clients and assist them in implementing their plan.

erinarian. Resources might also include pet loss support groups, human service agencies, church groups, and other animal-oriented organizations. The people associated with these groups usually don't have prior knowledge of your client and are usually only available during certain times. It may be helpful to encourage your client to identify and use as many different resources as possible.

After you have collected information about your clients' feelings and potential resources, you can help them create an action plan. The actual plan regarding how your client will get her needs met *must* come from the client herself. You may think you know the right path for your client to take or that you have the perfect solution for her problem; however, to ensure the plan's success, it is vital for the client to generate and adopt her own plan. This way, she will be more invested in the outcome and, if her plan fails, she can not blame you. Although you may think you know what is best in any given situation, *no one knows what is best for the client except the client!* Remember, unless it is morally, ethically, or professionally impossible to do so, you should support the decision your client makes.

Although you may think you know what is best in any given situation, no one knows what is best for the client except the client!

How Will I Know If I've Been Successful?

Communicating with clients on this level takes practice. At first, you may find yourself spending more time with clients than you want to and knowing more about their problems than you feel comfortable knowing. As you become more skilled at directing conversations, though, you'll find yourself capable of resolving complex emotional dilemmas in relatively short order in ways that are satisfying for you and your clients. You'll also develop a familiarity with your community's human and animal resources and become skilled at referring your clients to them.

Strategies:

Situation 4

Listening

Client: *I probably appear kind of crazy to you, worrying so much about a simple teeth cleaning, but I had another cat who died six years ago as a result of getting his teeth cleaned.*

What's Going on Here?

Pet owners come to your practices every day with a wide range of backgrounds and experiences. One of the simplest and most effective ways to connect and successfully communicate with a client is to develop good listening skills. Although listening sounds easy, it takes effort and practice to become a truly skilled listener.

Most of us are not taught to listen. During many conversations, it is not unusual for listeners to interrupt the speaker within the first several seconds. This is because, as listeners, we are more accustomed to interrupting people and to mentally preparing our next statements while someone is talking to us rather than to being attentive. The problem with not listening is that we miss out on valuable information the speaker is giving us. In your practice, resist the initial temptation to interrupt or ask your client a question right away. Try letting your clients speak for up to three minutes without interruption. This will set the stage for a solid connection between you.

> To listen in an active way, you simply focus on the emotional content of your client's message by tuning in to key "feeling" words or phrases and then giving your client permission to elaborate further on those feelings.

How Can I Connect?

Active listening means listening for feelings rather than for the factual content of conversations. This is a very powerful communication technique that can create deep connections between you and your clients. To listen in an active way, you simply focus on the emotional content of your client's message by tuning in to key "feeling" words or phrases and then giving your client permission to elaborate further on those feelings. Active listening is not problem solving. That comes later. Listening is the process of gathering information and insight into your client. Then, later, you can draw on these insights when your patient's medical condition requires you to support your client.

How Will I Know if I've Been Successful?

When you feel connected to your client and are communicating well, you will have listened skillfully. Most people are not accustomed to being listened to, so

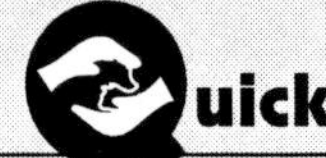

Quick Tips: What to Say, What to Do

- Structure the environment so it is conducive to listening. Remove as many barriers and distractions as possible. If you are on the telephone, don't try to do other things while you are speaking with a client.
- Use touch, attending behaviors, and active listening skills like minimal encouragers and silence to show clients you are following them.
- Approach the conversation with the right attitude. Your goal is to discover what your client thinks and feels. Be aware of your own physical and emotional status when listening. (Listening is difficult under conditions of fatigue, hunger, illness, or feeling upset, anxious, or preoccupied.)
- Paraphrase occasionally to let clients know you are listening:

  It sounds like you are feeling very worried about the teeth cleaning because of what happened to your other cat.
- Ask questions and use immediacy, gentle confrontation, and self-disclosure to move the conversation deeper to a more "feeling" level.
- Set appropriate and realistic boundaries. Some clients have so many questions and so much anxiety that you can't possibly meet their needs within your initial appointment time. Structure your time so that your interaction with the client can be productive, realistically fitting into the allotted time you have available for communication and for medicine. If a client needs to talk a lot and you have limited time, say something like, "It sounds like you have a lot going on and may need to talk more. I realize that I have limited time right now, but I could be available to you later in the day for about fifteen minutes to talk a bit more. Shall we schedule another fifteen minutes later at no additional charge to you?"

your clients will likely respond very positively and may bond very quickly to you if you have used good listening skills. Good listening doesn't need to take tremendous amounts of your time; it's the *quality* of your interaction that is the key. With the skillful use of active listening and paraphrasing, you can accomplish more in a five-minute conversation than you can in a twenty minute conversation with poor listening skills.

Strategies:

Situation 5

Body Language

Veterinarian 1 *(standing across the room from the client, shuffling papers, eyes downcast at the papers, speaking in a quiet, mumbling voice): The last estimate I gave you was about $100.00 too low. The actual cost of the treatment we discussed is $600.00.*

Client 1 *(arms crossed in front of her, eyes narrowed, brow furrowed, speaking in a loud voice, full of agitation): You better show me an itemized bill and be able to justify that added cost. I have a quote here in writing and I'm sure that, legally, I can hold you to this.*

Veterinarian 2 *(sitting on a chair next to the client, holding an itemized bill in front of both of them so they can both read it, smiling, using direct eye contact, and speaking in a voice that is clear, normally paced, and easily heard): Norma, I miscalculated on that first quote I gave you for Benson's treatment. As I looked at it more carefully, I realized I forgot to include the cost of the radiographs or x-rays. They are an additional $78.00. You can see here on the bill where I've added in that cost (pointing to the line on the bill). That brings the total cost of Benson's treatment to $598.35. Would you still like to proceed with the plan?*

Client 2 *(sitting next to the veterinarian, examining the itemized bill, body posture open, eyes wide, speaking in a normal voice): Yes, the additional cost presents a bit more of a problem for me, but I can see that it is necessary. Let's go ahead. I want to do whatever is best for Benson.*

What's Going On Here?

Body language is often called the silent language. Body language is composed of eye contact, facial expressions, hand gestures, and postures as well as the distance you put between you and another person. Clothes, hairstyles, colors, and jewelry are also part of body language.

Body language is often more believable than words because more than fifty percent of a message's impact is conveyed by it. The key to using body language successfully is congruence. Congruence means that the gestures, movements, eye contact, and facial expressions you use agree with or have the same meaning as the words you choose to use.

When your words and body language don't match, like in the opening scenario of this strategy, you send a confusing message to your listener. The result of this

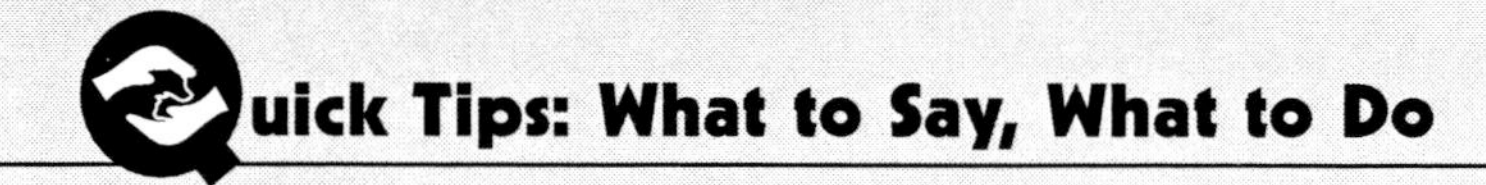

Quick Tips: What to Say, What to Do

- Structure the environment so you can sit or stand with an open body posture and make direct eye contact with your client. Remove or avoid putting physical barriers like desks or exam tables between you.
- Use hand movements and touch to direct your client's attention or to focus the conversation.
- Use attending behaviors to convey your willingness to listen to your client's point of view. Pay special attention to your own facial expressions as you listen, making sure they don't register thoughts or feelings that are incongruent with your verbal messages.
- Use active listening to explore your client's point of view. Pay special attention to how you use silences and minimal encouragers (head nods, eye blinks, smiles, etc.) to keep the conversation going.
- Monitor and control your voice tone, pitch, and pace. When dealing with someone's emotions, your voice should be pitched and paced a bit lower than normal as this is conveys comfort and concern.
- Use demonstrations and written materials to illustrate the verbal points you make.

confusion is usually mistrust, disbelief, misunderstanding, and even anger on the part of the listener.

How Can I Connect?

It's helpful to know the meanings of some of the typical gestures and body movements people make. Keep in mind, though, that the meanings of movements vary with genders, generations, cultures, and situations. For example, an older American woman who slouches and avoids eye contact may be expressing fatigue, depression, or a desire to not be noticed whereas a younger Puerto Rican man who slumps and avoids eye contact may be exhibiting signs of respect and deference to authority. The following list represents the most common meanings of several familiar body movements. The list is drawn from *How to Communicate: The Ultimate Guide to Improving Your Personal and Professional Relationships* by Matthew McKay, Martha Davis, and Patrick Fanning.

- ✔ smile = "I'm happy"
- ✔ frown and crossed arms = "I'm angry"
- ✔ drumming fingers = "I'm impatient"
- ✔ shrugged shoulders = "I don't care"
- ✔ heavy sigh = "I'm down"
- ✔ raised eyebrows = "I'm surprised"
- ✔ hand over mouth = "I'm horrified"
- ✔ furrowed forehead = "I'm concerned"
- ✔ wrinkled nose = "I don't like that"
- ✔ scratching the head = "I'm puzzled"
- ✔ rubbing the neck = "I'm frustrated or angry"

- ✔ touching the nose = "I doubt what you're (I'm) saying"
- ✔ tugging on an ear = "I want to interrupt"
- ✔ wringing hands together = "I'm sad, worried, grieving"
- ✔ rubbing hands together = "I'm anxious, excited"
- ✔ hands on knees = readiness
- ✔ hands or fingers on lips = impatience
- ✔ hands locked behind back = self-control
- ✔ hands locked behind head = a statement of superiority
- ✔ clenched fists = tension or anger
- ✔ arms extended out in front, palms out = sincerity
- ✔ arms crossed in front of chest = defensiveness
- ✔ sitting, straddling a chair = dominance
- ✔ sitting with one leg over the arm of a chair = indifference
- ✔ sitting with one ankle over the other knee or with ankles crossed = resistance
- ✔ sitting with one leg crossed over the other, swinging or kicking it back and forth = boredom, frustration
- ✔ rapid breathing = excitement, fear, anxiety, joy
- ✔ deep, slow breathing = relaxation, contentment

How Will I Know If I've Been Successful?

There is nothing more powerful than congruent communication. You will know when you are successfully using body language that matches your words because, overall, your communication with others will improve. You will notice that there are fewer misunderstandings between you and your clients, clients will be more likely to comply with your treatment recommendations, and your own conversational goals will be met more often. Your own status as a communicator may also change. If co-workers and clients previously viewed you as confusing and difficult to be around, they may now view you as someone who is easy to be around, easily understood, and skilled in the area of client relations. A welcome change!

The meanings of movements vary with genders, generations, cultures, and situations.

Strategies:

Situation 6

When You Must Say "No"

Client: *Dr. Meyer, I simply can't take any more time from work to bring Pepper in for his treatments. Can't you make an exception for me and see me in the evening, after dinner? I could be at your office promptly at seven.*

What's Going On Here?

Occasionally, clients make requests that you either can't or don't want to grant. If you're like the majority of other caring veterinarians, you probably find yourself saying "yes" to your clients more often than "no," even though saying "yes" makes you feel angry and resentful.

Of course, most veterinarians would rather have their clients' approval than not have their approval. However, if you have a hard time saying no to clients (especially when saying no is completely appropriate!), the need to gain *everyone's* approval *all of the time* may be a significant problem for you. The problem occurs when saying yes to a client results in you neglecting your own needs or the needs of your family or friends. For example, if you agree to see Pepper at 7:00 because you fear losing your client's approval or business, you neglect your own needs (instead of eating a nutritious meal with your family, you go next door for a taco) as well as your family's needs (you miss a planned family event at your child's school).

When it comes to effective communication, then, one of the most important techniques you can learn is how to say no. Saying no allows you to set limits and maintain the boundaries between your personal and professional lives. Maintaining appropriate boundaries also preserves your energy and enthusiasm and prevents you from experiencing professional "burn-out."

> The desire to be all things to all people is overwhelming. It often results in confusing communication and in taking on more than can be comfortably managed.

How Can I Connect?

The desire to be all things to all people is overwhelming. It often results in confusing communication and in taking on more than can be comfortably managed. Thus, setting boundaries not only improves communication, it can also help maintain your sanity.

A boundary is a pre-determined or pre-established limit. A boundary establishes a guideline regarding your flexibility. Everyone has personal and professional boundaries or limits that regulate their behaviors and their responses to others. The problem is that most of us are unaware of our boundaries.

Skilled communicators need to acknowledge their boundaries and give themselves permission to persistently abide by them. When boundaries and priorities are clearly defined and openly discussed, others know

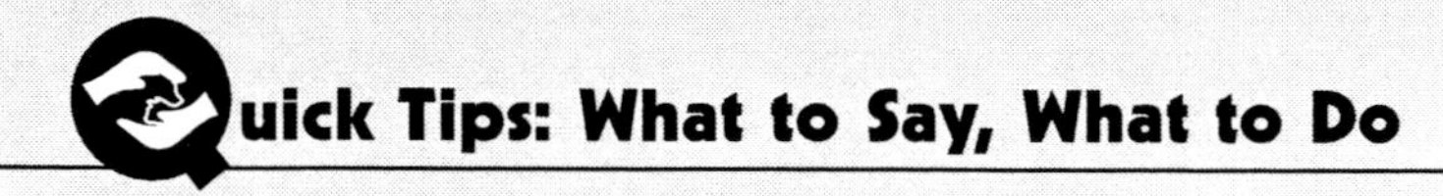

Quick Tips: What to Say, What to Do

- Acknowledge your client's need or request and clearly establish your limits:

  I understand it's difficult to ask for time away from your job; however, I don't make appointments during the evening hours.

- Use self-disclosure to solidify or to justify your limits (if you feel you must):

  As I said, I don't make evening appointments. I have a spouse and two young children who are my priorities after work.

- If the client persists, use immediacy or gentle confrontation to repeat your "no" answer and maintain your boundaries:

  You and Pepper are important to me and I respect the fact that you need to make arrangements to have Pepper treated at a time when it won't interfere with your job. However, I'm beginning to feel frustrated with your unwillingness to understand and accommodate my schedule.

- Say no to the request you can not grant, but offer a compromise:

  I can't see you at seven at night, but you can drop Pepper off before eight and pick him up at five. We'll treat him and care for him while you're at work.

- As the conversation proceeds, use attending, direct eye contact, active listening, paraphrasing, and touch to ensure that your non-verbal behaviors reinforce your words. If you are talking to your client on the telephone, pay special attention to the tone of your voice.
- Provide your client with written materials stating your clinic's policies regarding treatment schedules, appointment hours, after-hours emergency fees, etc.

what to expect. For example, when you tell your clients and co-workers that your family is your first priority and that, with the exception of true emergencies, you will not see patients after 5:00 p.m., they will be more likely to respect your boundaries and support you when you must say no.

How Will I Know If I've Been Successful?

You will know you are successfully setting limits and saying no appropriately when you enjoy your job instead of resenting it. Your friends and family will also be indicators of success because they will stop feeling disappointed and neglected and will feel they finally get to spend enough time with you. Even though you may occasionally lose a demanding client who cannot deal with your boundaries and firm refusals, the majority of your clients will understand, respect, and approve of your priorities and be more than willing to negotiate mutually acceptable compromises.

Strategies:

Situation 7

Indecisive Clients

Amy: *I just don't know if I should go ahead with Max's surgery. I know that it's risky to do it, but I also know that it is Max's only real chance. I don't think I'm ready to let him go yet without trying something, but I'm just so confused. Dr. Prescott, what would you do if Max were your dog?*

Veterinarian: *Amy, I can see how difficult this decision is for you. You want to give Max every chance possible yet there are no guarantees. The fact is that what I might do for Max if he were my dog and what you might choose to do could be very different. There really is not a right or wrong answer here. But, Amy, the most important thing for you to know is that, whichever decision you make, I'll support you all the way.*

What's Going on Here?

Pet owners face difficult decisions every day. Clients who care deeply for their animals often struggle with decisions about procedures like surgery, amputation, chemotherapy, and euthanasia. Since companion animals are almost completely dependent upon their owners for their care and well-being, many owners feel that they have made unspoken "contracts" with their animals to love and take care of them. This sense of responsibility can create great emotional distress for owners when they believe that their animals are trusting them with their lives.

The single most important thing to discuss with indecisive clients is the issue of quality of life for the animal. This will give you and the client a common reference point and a way of structuring your interaction. Different clients have different standards for quality of life and each may define it in unique ways, according to the individual personality of the owner and the animal. Your job is to help clients identify their definition of what quality of life means for their animals and to communicate that you understand this. This might mean accepting a definition for quality of life that is somewhat different than your own.

How Can I Connect?

Indecisiveness usually stems from anxiety and a need to make the "right" decision. During decision-making, then, your goal is to help clients realize that there may not be a "right" decision, only a decision that is right for them. The other part of your job is to lower your clients' anxiety about the decision-making process, normalizing their feelings within the context of their love for their animal. Some other helpful decision-making techniques are:

- **Ask if clients need more medical information.**
  Would it be helpful if we reviewed the surgery once again and discussed the potential side effects?
- **Help clients look at future consequences and potential circumstances.**
  When you look back on this six months from now, Amy, what will be most important about what you did

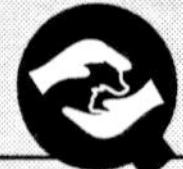

Quick Tips: What to Say, What to Do

- Normalize your client's feelings and self-disclose, if appropriate:

  I know how much Max means to you and I can tell what a difficult decision this is for you. I would be struggling as much as you are if I were in your shoes.

- Acknowledge your client's unique relationship with her companion animal:

  You and Max have a very special relationship and you are the expert on what is best for him. I can give you my medical opinions, but the fact is, I don't know him and understand him the way that you do.

- Give your client permission to feel anxious and re-frame it as a positive trait:

  Given how much you love Max, I'd be worried about you if you weren't struggling with this decision. The fact that you are having trouble making a decision about his surgery is a sign of how much you truly care about him and want what is best.

- If there is no medical reason to require an immediate decision, structure the environment in a way that gives your client access to a private room and a telephone so she can think and consult with friends or family members, and remove time barriers so she can take several hours or even days to make the decision:

  Amy, it seems like you're not 100 percent sure about your decision. Since there is no medical reason to rush, would you like to take Max home and give yourself some more time to prepare?

- Once a decision has been made, paraphrase your client's words and feelings to ensure you are both committed to the same course of action:

  It sounds like you want to proceed with Max's surgery. I understand that you feel anxious about it, and I also hear that you feel you would not forgive yourself if you did not give Max this chance. Am I hearing you correctly?

or did not do? Which decisions will be the easiest for you to live with? I believe it's part of my job to help you make decisions now that will keep your regrets minimal later on.

- **Encourage clients to "talk" with their animals.** Many owners have very special relationships with their pets. When tough decisions need to be made, you can encourage your clients to enlist their pets' help with their decisions:

Amy, you and Max have always been able to communicate with one another. That is still the case now. Spend some time with Max, talk to him, and maybe he will be able to tell you what he wants. Based on how strongly connected the two of you are, I believe that you will come to the answer that is right for you together.

- **Be open to discussing euthanasia as an option if the medical status of the animal warrants it.** Be aware that clients might not want to pursue treatment but may be hesitant to tell you because they don't want to look like a bad or uncaring person:

Amy, we know that Max's cancer is quite advanced. We've discussed options for treatment, but I want you to know that euthanasia is also an option. Doing every possible treatment for Max is not necessarily proof of how much you love him. Looking at his quality of life is also a sign of your love and I want you to know that I will also support that decision if it's the one you come to.

Different clients have different standards for quality of life and each may define it in a unique way, according to the individual personality of the owner and the animal.

How Will I Know if I've Been Successful?

When clients make decisions that are best for their animals and themselves, you will know that you have been an effective communicator. While you might not always agree with your clients' decisions, you will have the satisfaction of knowing that you connected with them during an emotionally tough time and used several communication techniques to truly help them.

Strategies:

___

___

___

___

___

___

___

___

___

___

___

Situation 8

Resolving Differences and Misunderstandings with Clients

Client: *I think I'm going to take Schroeder to another veterinary clinic. I'm tired of the indifferent attitude around here. You said you'd call me at eleven and it's now two fifteen! I don't have the time to wait by the phone all day!*

Veterinarian: *I hear that you're frustrated and unhappy with the care you've received lately, Mary. Schroeder is a great dog and deserves the best. I believe I did say I would call you at eleven unless I had surgeries to perform. In that case, I recall telling you that I may not be able to talk to until around two.*

Client: *I don't remember you saying that. All I heard was eleven!*

Veterinarian: *I apologize if I didn't make that clear, Mary. I hate to be kept waiting, too, especially when I'm worried about someone I love. As it turned out, I did have an emergency surgery and I didn't finish until a short time ago. Can we spend a few minutes now talking about Schroeder's condition?*

What's Going on Here?

Most conflicts result from miscommunication. They often start small, with very minor issues, and escalate into full-blown conflicts. The key to resolving conflict successfully is to identify at which point in time you and your client might have miscommunicated and then begin to clear up any and all misunderstandings that arose from that time. If left unresolved, simple misunderstandings, like confusion over when you will call a client back, can create hurt feelings and lead to larger problems down the road. Left unresolved, misunderstandings can also lead to the erroneous assumption that you don't care about your clients.

Behind most conflicts, you will find clients whose feelings are hurt in some way. They may feel hurt because they feel you ignored their needs, trivialized their problems, or ridiculed their emotions. If you can find out *why* your clients feel hurt, you can usually get to the heart of the matter and work things out.

The single most important factor in successful conflict resolution is your attitude and willingness to work through the problem. If you demonstrate a sincere desire to resolve the problem (both through your words and your non-verbal behavior) you can actually enhance and improve your relationship with an unhappy client. Some clients may actually respect you more after a conflict because you have shown a keen interest in them by being an open, honest, and a skilled communicator.

How Can I Connect?

Conflict resolution is an advanced communication technique that can be developed over time. The first barrier most communicators need to get past is their initial

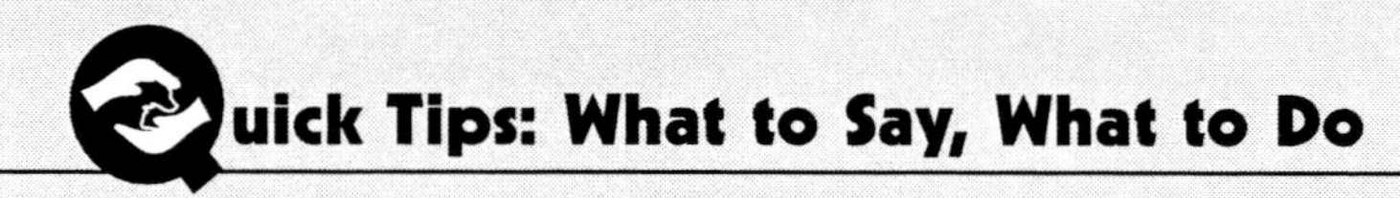

Quick Tips: What to Say, What to Do

- Acknowledge your client's feelings:

  It sounds like you're unhappy with the way we've treated you.

- Structure the environment and invite your client to talk with you more in a private, quiet area:

  Would you be willing to come with me to my office so that we could talk more about this?

- If the conversation is taking place on the telephone, tell your client you want to move to a more private telephone and ask for permission to put her on hold for a few moments.

- Use open-ended questions to identify your client's needs, problems, complaints, or concerns:

  Can you tell me exactly what happened that brought us to this point?

- Use active listening and paraphrasing to ensure that you understand your client's point of view and that you are reaching some common ground for further discussion.

- Use open, attending behavior to lend credibility to your words. If you tell your client that you want to understand but convey defensiveness or lack of concern with your non-verbal behavior, your client will not believe a word you say.

- Self-disclose about a time when you might have been in a similar situation:

  I hate to be kept waiting, too, especially when I'm worried about someone I love.

- If necessary, use gentle confrontation to communicate your point of view and to set limits. It might be necessary to re-educate your client about clinic policies, surgery schedules, or the details of your previous conversations.

- Use immediacy to summarize and end the conversation, thanking your client for their willingness to work through the problem:

  Thank you for taking the time to help me figure out where we got off track. I feel much better now that we've talked and I'm looking forward to seeing you and Schroeder again.

reluctance or fear of "getting into it" when there is a client-relations problem. It's often easier to dismiss clients' complaints as "their problems" and to blame them for causing "unnecessary" turmoil. Some veterinarians even prefer to lose clients to other veterinary practices rather than subject themselves to the conflict resolution process.

Most clients, though, are impressed by veterinarians who are confident and willing to talk about tough issues. Confidence is your most powerful tool. Remind yourself that most conflicts can be traced back to a fairly simple misunderstanding and that you can accomplish a great deal toward resolving a client-relations conflict if you proceed step-by-step toward unraveling the problem.

Many of us are taught that conflict is about "winning" and "losing." Rather, it is about improving communication. When attempting to resolve a conflict with a client, it's more helpful to view the interaction as an opportunity for enhanced understanding between the two of you, rather than viewing the conversation as a chance to fight it out. The goal is for both of you to get your needs met and to find some form of compromise or solution to the problem. During a busy day, the extra fifteen minutes that you take for conflict resolution might mean the difference between losing a client's business forever or retaining her as a loyal client for many years to come.

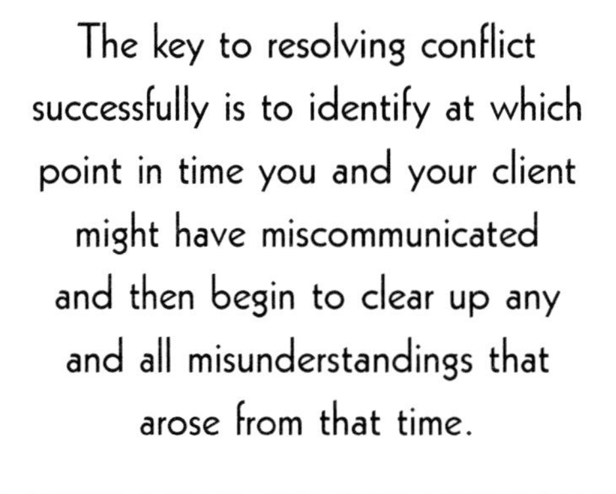

How Will I Know if I've Been Successful?

Your client's continuing business will let you know. Many people who find ways to successfully work through conflict also feel a sense of personal gratification in knowing that they worked through a tough issue and gained positive results.

Another indicator might be a greater level of job satisfaction for you. Many veterinarians report that one of the major sources of stress and burn-out is dealing with client conflicts and the residual feelings of frustration and resentment that unresolved conflicts leave behind.

It is important to note that these principles apply to resolving conflicts that occur among your staff and employees as well. Positive conflict management with your co-workers is just as critical, if not more, as it is with your clients. Regular staff meetings can be an excellent forum to address conflicts and to provide time for working through them.

Strategies:

Situation 9

When You Need to Apologize

Mark and Sophia Taylor choose cremation for their dog Pooch after he dies. They wish to have Pooch individually cremated with the remains returned to them afterwards. Since your clinic offers this service to clients, you agree to make the appropriate arrangements with the local pet cemetery/crematory.

After a week, you realize that Pooch's remains have not come back to your office. After speaking with the people at the crematory and checking back through your own records, you realize that you forgot to write down your clients' request for individual cremation. The pet crematory's policy is that, without written instructions designating a body for individual cremation, all bodies are taken care of by mass cremation with the remains scattered on the grounds of the pet cemetery. The sick feeling in your stomach tells you that this is what happened to Pooch.

You know how upsetting this news will be for the Taylors. It occurs to you that, rather than telling the Taylors the truth, it might be kinder to scoop us some remains at the pet crematory, give them to the Taylors, and let them think they belonged to Pooch. Or you might tell them that the crematory lost their paperwork and didn't bother to call you to see what arrangements the Taylors had made.

You're concerned about protecting yourself. Perhaps you shouldn't admit your mistake. What if the Taylors take their business to another clinic or, even worse, decide to sue you?

You decide to spare the Taylors any further pain and give them remains that are not Pooch's. However, you neglect to update your co-workers about your plan. On the day the Taylors pick up Pooch's remains, one of your co-workers sees them as they are leaving. She sincerely offers her condolences on Pooch's death and also mentions how sorry she is about the mix-up with the cremations. Confused, the Taylors return to you and ask for an honest explanation.

What's Going On Here?

Honesty respects the truth. However, in the world of medicine (both human and veterinary), honesty can be a controversial ethical principle. Most everyone agrees that there is a "rightness" to telling the truth. However, since veterinarians are committed to working for the *benefit* of their patients and clients, some are skeptical about telling the truth "for truth's sake." As in the opening scenario, when there is a seemingly harmless opportunity to correct a mistake, telling the truth often seems to create more harm than good. However, if

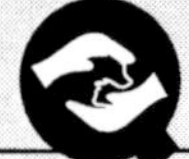

Quick Tips: What to Say, What to Do

- Structure your environment so you have a quiet, private, comfortable place to talk.
- Acknowledge your mistake, delivering the news in a sensitive way.
- Use active listening and paraphrasing to understand your clients' responses and current requests.
- Be immediate with your own feelings, self-disclose about your own feelings of sadness and regret.

you take time to think through the possible consequences brought on by a seemingly harmless lie (lawsuits, loss of business, serious damage to your reputation and credibility), a strong case for honesty can be built.

Being honest goes hand-in-hand with being willing and able to apologize when you have made a mistake. To apologize is to express regret. In some cases, offering an apology also means taking responsibility and attempting to "right" a "wrong." When you decide to be honest and to apologize to a client, it is an opportunity to use every communication technique described in this book. While apologizing and being honest are almost always the professional and the "right" thing to do, it takes tremendous courage for you to do so!

How Can I Connect?

Some people refuse to apologize, even when they know they are clearly wrong, because they don't want to feel like they're in a vulnerable position. For them, being vulnerable usually feels like a loss of power or strength. Some people blame others when mistakes are made. Blaming is a way to shirk responsibility and to cast others as the ones who are at fault. Psychologists say we blame others for things we've done because we are afraid of rejection and afraid that people will think less of us if they find out what we've done. Still others apologize and take responsibility for everything that goes wrong, even when they are clearly *not* responsible. None of these attitudes are effective ways to communicate or effective ways to rectify mistakes.

There is an effective communication strategy for offering an apology. It's based on a model for delivering bad news that has been proven to be more effective than other models. The model is a three-step one: 1) prepare clients emotionally for what is to come, 2) predict how clients may feel or respond when the news is given, and 3) proceed to offer clients information in brief conversations. For instance, you might cover steps one and two by saying:

> *Mr. and Mrs. Taylor, I have some bad news that may be upsetting for you to hear.*

followed by:

> *When Pooch died, I said I would be responsible for making the arrangements to have him cremated. After*

you left, I filled out the form for the crematory, but I neglected to note your wishes concerning individual cremation and the return of Pooch's remains. As a result, Pooch was part of a mass cremation and I am unable to give you his individual remains. I sincerely apologize. I am so sorry I made this mistake.

After saying this much, stop and attend to your clients' emotional reactions. Prepare yourself for anything—sobbing, cries of disbelief, anger, or even complete silence. Once your clients' initial reactions have passed, ask what they need next. Some choices might include providing them with more detailed information now or setting an appointment to speak with them again later in the day. You may also want to offer to connect them directly with the pet crematory so they can resolve this dilemma in their own way.

Being honest goes hand-in-hand with being willing and able to apologize when you have made a mistake.

How Will I Know if I've Been Successful?

Your honesty and willingness to apologize will pay off when your clients forgive you and remain loyal to your practice. You will also know you have been successful when the feelings of trust, rapport, and respect between you and your clients deepen.

However, even if you encounter clients who refuse to forgive you and take their business elsewhere, it's important for you to acknowledge that there is personal success in simply doing the "right" thing, regardless of the outcome. Congratulations!

Strategies:

___

___

___

___

___

___

___

___

___

___

___

Situation 10

Humor

Veterinarian: *. . . and that's the "Big Picture" regarding Molly's treatment over the next six weeks, Tina. I know I've given you a lot of details and the appointment schedule we've mapped out may seem overwhelming. If you decide to go through with it, though, I believe Molly has a very good chance for complete recovery.*

So . . . shall we start Molly's first treatment today or do you want to bring her back first thing tomorrow morning?

Client: *(stunned silence)*

Veterinarian: *(touching Tina's arm to get her attention, making direct eye contact, smiling, and using a soft, understanding voice) Tina, if you answer this question correctly, you might win the trip to Cabo San Lucas!*

Client: *(shakes her head, makes eye contact, and giggles) Well, with this treatment schedule, how in the world can I go on a vacation?*

What's Going On Here?

Consider a typical morning at your clinic. Everything runs smoothly until about 10:00. Then, two clients arrive late for their appointments and throw off your schedule. Clients begin to "stack up" in your waiting area. A client who has just been seen by you has questions about the charges on her bill. While you are consulting with her, one of your long-term clients calls and says he has a very sick dog whom he feels can't be moved. He wonders if you could come to his home as soon as possible. During your conversation with him, a woman bursts through your front door with a cat who has been hit by a car and a delivery man arrives with several heavy crates of pet food that need to be signed for and moved out of the waiting room to your storeroom.

Veterinary medicine is a demanding profession. During a typical work day, you solve complex medical problems, provide medical treatment, attend to business details, and provide emotional support for your clients. Stress—for both you and your clients—is inevitable, and stress can significantly affect communication.

Sometimes humor is "just what the doctor ordered" to reduce rising tension levels and restore balance to situations that are beginning to escalate out of control. As long as the humor pokes fun at the situation and not at the people involved, a well-placed, funny comment can go a long way toward building rapport and meeting your client's need to "lighten up." Remember, laughter *is* often the best medicine.

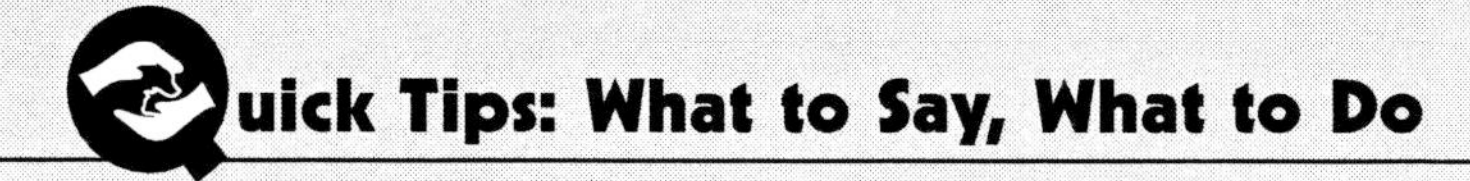

Quick Tips: What to Say, What to Do

- Acknowledge the irony, tension, or difficulty of a situation in an unexpected, unpredictable way. When used as an effective communication strategy, humor should be victimless. For example, in response to the choas described in the opening scenario, the veterinarian might make a comment like, "I'll be back to take care of all of these people as soon as I finish painting my office!"
- Use humor to normalize your client's situation:

  You know, Tina, every dog I talk to in my office tells me the same thing..."My mom and dad are worriers, so you're going to have to help them through this frightening time."
- Use humor when you use props, offer written materials, or demonstrate a procedure to your clients. When it's not a matter of life or death, one veterinarian always refers to radiographs as "the Halloween version of your pet" and draws silly cartoon caricatures of his patients on any written materials he provides for owners. Many veterinary practices send humorous reminders when it's time for a pet's check-up, vaccination, etc.
- Self-disclose about your own particular brand of humor and use immediacy if you feel your attempt to be funny may have hurt or offended your client.

  Tina, I'm aware that my sense of humor is a bit cynical at times. I noticed the expression on your face changed just now. Did I say something that offended you?
- If you're not laughing enough, take a humor break during the most tense part of your day. Keep a humor file of cartoons, pictures, and jokes or spend time with people or animals who make you laugh.

How Can I Connect?

Both research and clinical experience show that, when stress and tension levels are high, people often stop even attempting to communicate well. The unconscious belief is that effective communication takes too much effort and that, during tense times, the priorities are keeping schedules on-track and accomplishing the multitude of tasks that need to be done.

However, this attitude often creates more stress in the forms of client complaints, hurt feelings, and misunderstandings. When you set aside effective communication techniques, it's like performing a surgical procedure with a butter knife and a knitting needle. You're going to do some damage. If high stress levels cause you to withdraw, become distracted, or avoid dealing with the emotional content of certain conversations, you're likely to be viewed as more abrupt, flippant, sarcastic, and uncaring. During times of stress, thoughtless comments and behaviors are often misinterpreted by clients.

Humor is a remedy for stress. Instead of withdrawing or abruptly barking orders at those around you, try making them laugh instead. Laughter is a great tension reliever. A good laugh gives the heart muscles a workout, improves circulation, clears the respiratory passages, stimulates alertness hormones, diminishes tension in the central nervous system, counteracts fear, anger, and depression, and possibly relieves pain.

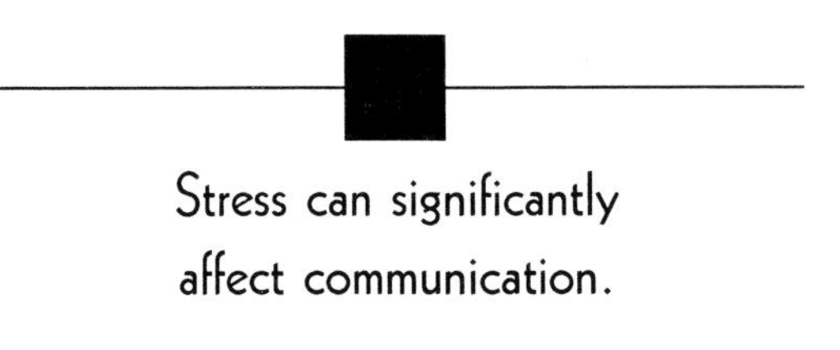

Stress can significantly affect communication.

However, remember that men and women tend to use and respond to different types of humor. While it's more common for men to tease, playfully insult each other, or make mock verbal attacks on one another, it's more common for women to mock themselves. These style differences are often misunderstood by the opposite gender, with women taking men's playful insults seriously and feeling offended by them and men viewing women's self-deprecating humor as evidence of their low self-esteem and uncertainty. Age, cultural background, educational level, religious orientation, political affiliation, and a myriad of other variables can also affect how humor is viewed. However, while humor should be used cautiously, it should be used!

While it's probably not enough to just tell yourself to be funny, contrary to most peoples' beliefs, humor can be learned. Pay attention to those around you who seem to be naturally funny. What lines do they use over and over? When do they insert humorous comments into conversations? Use funny people as role models and allow yourself to try out some of their techniques.

How Will I Know if I've Been Successful?

People who have a well-developed sense of humor tend to be thought of as more creative, flexible, open, and approachable. People who use humor are often sought out by others because it feels good to be around them. You'll know you're using humor effectively when your clients return to your practice and tell you how much they enjoy their visits with you. Watch your clients' faces. If they're smiling and laughing with you, you're probably on the right track.

Strategies:

Situation 11

Complaining or Demanding Clients

Client: *I'm very disappointed in the way Winston was treated at your hospital. When I brought him home, he had a foul odor and looked tired. He was upset for two whole days and I had a difficult time coaxing him to come out of the bedroom. What in the world happened to him when he was with you?*

What's Going on Here?

Like many professionals providing a service to the public, veterinarians have to deal with client complaints and demands. Even though your profession is about medicine, you are still in a business that requires customer satisfaction. In veterinary medicine, client complaints and demands can range from the predictable and expected, to the outrageous and unreasonable. Many factors can determine how demanding or satisfied a given client will be. These include: client personality, client expectations (realistic vs. unrealistic), the bond between the client and animal, and the client's perceptions of veterinary care. Complaints and demands are a regular part of your practice. The key is how you respond to these situations. Your most powerful tool is your ability to communicate well with your client. If you can do this, you will save yourself valuable amounts of time and tons of frustration.

How Can I Connect?

Pet owners can feel very scared and powerless when their animals become sick, especially when they don't have the power to make their loved ones feel better. Therefore, they look to you to help them. In order to allow you to help their pet, they must withdraw their own control and place their trust in you. This can make owners feel very vulnerable. A person attempting to cope with feelings of fear and helplessness can become very demanding or critical. Sometimes complaining about your services or demanding special treatment is a way for clients to "test" you (get your attention, regain some control) and to "keep you on your toes." They might deduce that, if you are able to handle their complaints and meet every demand they throw at you, you are probably also capable of successfully treating their companion animal. Most clients don't consciously decide to behave this way. Rather, their complaints and demands are unconscious reactions to their feelings of anxiety. While it's true that most clients cannot accurately assess your medical skills, they can certainly assess your communication skills. Thus, you can mitigate a lot of complaints and demands by simply acknowledging your clients' feelings and gently reassuring them that you care.

You can be proactive and often prevent client complaints by providing good client education. For instance, you should always prepare clients for any potential complications, problems, appearances, or behaviors that might be of concern after a medical procedure or surgery:

Kim, when we bring Winston to you I want you to be aware that he will look differently than when you left him here yesterday. He has an incision on his belly that is about three inches long. We shaved the fur around this area and there is a bandage covering the incision. This area might be red and swollen for a day or two. He might also smell a bit funny from the anesthesia and have some spots on his fur. Also, Winston might not be his usual bouncy self for a few days. This is normal after a surgery and will give him time to rest and recuperate.

I have written down some instructions for you on how to take care of him and what to look for if there are complications. If you think of any other concerns, please call us during our office hours and we'd be glad to help you.

You and your co-workers are a team when it comes to working with overly demanding clients. It's important to ensure that you are all communicating the same message. Be careful to set limits up front and don't let clients "split" your staff. For example, if one member of your staff gets intimidated and bends the rules to accommodate a demanding client, it will be difficult for someone else to set limits later on and to enforce clinic policies. Remember to work together to try to meet your client's needs while also supporting each other.

A person attempting to cope with feelings of fear and helplessness can become very demanding or critical.

How Will I Know if I've Been Successful?

A satisfied client will tell you whether or not you have been successful in working through any complaints or demands. Except in the rare cases when you have completely unreasonable clients (and there are some), you can usually address complaints and demands with good communication. As mentioned earlier, pet owners will probably not know when you have practiced good medicine, but they will certainly know when you have made them feel cared about, reassured, and understood. As you are in a business that competes for "customers", it is important not to underestimate the value of good communication. If you are perceived as a skilled communicator, there's every chance that your clients will also perceive you as a skilled veterinarian.

Strategies:

____

____

____

____

____

____

____

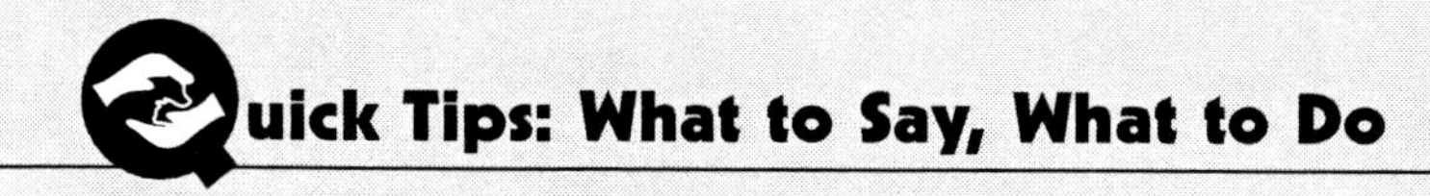

Quick Tips: What to Say, What to Do

- Recognize that complaining or demanding clients may be highly bonded to their animals and feeling very anxious or worried about their pets. Take time to determine the exact nature of your client's needs, problems, complaints, or concerns:

  I hear that you are very concerned about Winston and want him to have the very best care possible. Let's go over your concerns one-by-one and see if we can clear up any doubts that you may have regarding the care we provided.

- Use open-ended questions to determine what is motivating the client to complain or to be demanding:

  What is your biggest concern at this point?

  What could we have done differently?

  Can you tell me more about what you're thinking or feeling?

  How can I best support you through this?

  Where would you like to go from here?

- Acknowledge your client's complaints and invite her to discuss them with you further. Don't get defensive in response, but rather open the lines of communication by actively listening to what she has to say. You can then evaluate whether or not the complaint seems justified or unreasonable.

- *If the complaint seems justified,* you may want to apologize and adjust your care to fit the client's needs. Client education regarding your view as to the cause of the misunderstanding may also be useful.

  I'm sorry you had to wait an hour past your scheduled appointment today. We had an emergency this morning that needed our immediate attention in order to save the animal's life. We appreciate your patience and in the future we will notify you of changes in our appointment schedules. As for today, would you like me to examine Buddy now or would you like to reschedule?

- *If the complaint seems unreasonable,* acknowledge the client's feelings while setting limits and providing client education.

  I can see that you had hoped to be seen immediately today and that you are concerned about Casey. Unfortunately, we can't always respond to a walk-in appointment right away. Since Casey's condition isn't critical, I need to see the four other clients who had scheduled appointments first. I can either see you and Casey as soon as I'm finished with them or you can make an appointment with the receptionist for another time.

- Overly demanding clients may have unrealistic expectations of you and your co-workers. Ask questions that will help you to determine how realistic their expectations are:

  Mrs. Baker, what are your expectations of me and of our staff?

  What is your goal in coming here today?

  I can see that you had different ideas about how your appointment with Winston would go today. Let me share with you how our hospital works and answer any questions that you might have to see if we can meet your needs.

- If you get stuck, always acknowledge the bond between the animal and owner. Ask your client to work with you to address the complaint.

  I know that you are unhappy at this point and I'm not sure if we're getting anywhere. It's so obvious to me that Winston is very important to you and it's important to me that you and Winston receive quality care. Can you help me figure out what we could do together to resolve our differences and continue to help Winston?

Situation 12

Fearful and Anxious Clients

Client: *I don't know what to do for Milton. I want him to feel better, but I'm afraid to treat him! I'm so afraid that something awful will happen to him!*

What's Going on Here?

It is challenging to communicate with and support clients who are feeling anxious, fearful, or out of control. As discussed in earlier strategies, it is natural for clients to have these feelings when their animals are ill or injured, and they are relying on you to know what to do to help them. Most pet owners entrust the care of their animals to you without having much medical knowledge to accurately evaluate your skills. Some clients will express their fears openly, while others might express their anxiety in disguised ways, like being overly demanding, suspicious, or even hostile.

The best way to help fearful or anxious clients is to acknowledge their feelings and to normalize their emotions. Most people find it reassuring to know that what they are thinking and feeling is to be expected.

Creating a trusting and positive working relationship takes time, effort, and patience.

How Can I Connect?

Most pet owners who worry while their animals are being treated have two primary questions: 1) "Is my animal in any pain?" and 2) "Is there anyone with my animal?" These two fundamental fears—that the animal is hurting and that the animal is alone—can be addressed by your thoughtful communication. Some strategies that might be helpful are to:

- **paint a comforting visual image for clients.**
  Clients who are overly anxious might create frightening or distressing images of their pets' circumstances unless you replace their false image with a more accurate one.

  Tim, right now Milton is waking up from his surgery. He's lying comfortably on a big, soft blanket and my technician Christy is petting him and talking to him. He'll stay with us throughout the day so that we can monitor his progress and watch him very closely. We've given him some pain medication and he'll likely feel drowsy for a while. It looks like Christy and Milton have taken a liking to each other. She seems to have found a certain spot on his chest that he particularly likes to have rubbed. I'm sure that he'll be getting a lot of attention until you come to take him home tonight.

- **provide tours of your facility to help reassure clients.**
  Clients who are distrustful or fearful of medical facilities can imagine that outrageous procedures take place in your "back rooms" even though they may not openly share these fears with you. During a tour, you can convey trustworthiness and

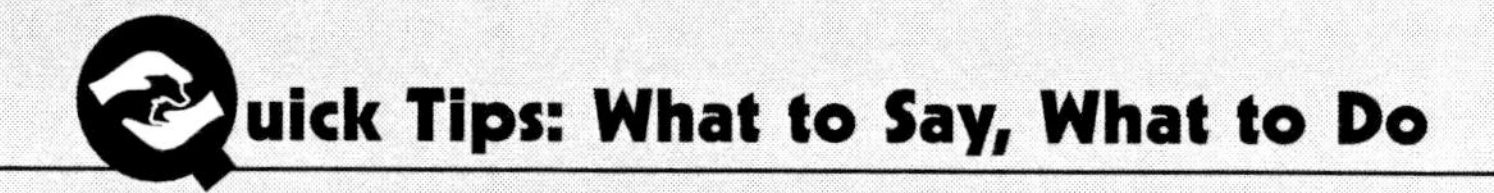

Quick Tips: What to Say, What to Do

- Acknowledge your client's feelings
- Normalize your client's feelings in the context of his relationship with his animal:

  Tim, given how much you care about Milton, it would be strange if you weren't anxious about his surgery.
- Self-disclose about your own emotions, if you feel it is appropriate:

  I love my dog, too, and think of her as part of my family. If I were in your shoes and she was about to have surgery, I'd also be worried and scared.
- Ask open-ended questions to find out how you might assist the client:

  How can I best support you with this?

  What would be most helpful for you right now?
- Use gentle confrontation when the client's anxiety or fear prevents them from making a decision or taking action when immediate action is needed.

  Tim, I know that this is a very difficult situation for you and that you don't want to have to think about this now. Unfortunately, Milton's medical status requires that we take action as soon as possible. What can I provide for you that will help you make your decision?

warmth by showing clients that you are not "hiding" anything from them. Of course, it's a good idea to prepare your co-workers before you bring clients through your treatment and surgery areas.

How Will I Know if I've Been Successful?

When you have calmed clients' anxieties and helped them face their fears, it will usually become easier to communicate with them. Creating a trusting and positive working relationship takes time, effort, and patience. You might not always be able to completely eliminate your clients' fears, but for many pet owners, a little reassurance is all they need.

Strategies:

Situation 13

Angry Clients

Client: *I'm not going to pay a cent for this surgery! Wally is sicker now that when I first brought him in to see you. I really wonder if any of you know what you're doing around here and if any of you really give a damn about him at all!*

What's Going on Here?

Pet owners become angry for a variety of reasons and can express their anger in various ways. Anger is a difficult emotion to deal with because of the negative energy it creates and the negative responses it illicits. Some typical reasons why pet owners become angry are:

- **Finances**
  an inability to pay or unrealistic expectations about the cost of veterinary services
- **Treatment complications and unexpected problems**
- **Dissatisfaction with services**
  the perception that their animal has been mishandled or mistreated in some way
- **Time conflicts**
  unrealistic expectations as to time involved; being kept waiting
- **Poor communication**
  minor misunderstandings, unresolved conflicts
- **Lack of information/Lack of preparation**
  not being informed of a pet's condition or treatment, feeling inadequately prepared to deal with a pet's illness (physical appearance, financial issues, future problems) or death
- **Lack of continuity of care**
  seeing a different veterinarian during each visit, feeling "passed around"
- **Emotional responses to an animal's illness or death**
  some people use anger as a mask for other emotions they are feeling as a result of a pet's illness or death; anger is sometimes expressed because it is easy to access. Typical emotions that are often masked by anger include helplessness, powerlessness, fear, guilt, sadness, and grief.

How Can I Connect?

Anger is a normal, natural emotion that all people feel. What makes anger so difficult for most people to deal with is the negative energy behind it. If you work to understand why your client is angry, you have a much better chance at diffusing it. The key is to stay calm and try to keep the situation under control.

There are, of course, times when another person's anger is abusive or completely inappropriate. In these situations, your job is to protect yourself and your staff. Your responsibility as a care provider never extends to remaining in a place or near a person that is abusive or potentially dangerous.

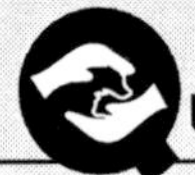

Quick Tips: What to Say, What to Do

- Know your own responses to anger. Some people "freeze up" when confronted with intense anger while others tend to lash back. Know your own "anger buttons" and be aware of how and when clients might push those buttons. Take a few deep breaths to calm your body and gain your composure. While you are breathing, think about ways that you can *respond* to the anger rather than *react* to it.
- Don't get defensive. The majority of people who are angry just want to be heard and understood. A client's anger is usually more about her own frustrations or problems than it is about you. If you take it personally and lose your cool, you will only escalate the level of anger. Help the person regain control and model this for them by staying in control yourself. Remember that, in reality, the more powerful person is the relaxed one.
- Let your client "vent." Once a client has blown off steam, they can more easily discuss the issue rationally.
- Move your discussion to a private place and structure your environment so you can calmly speak face-to-face.
- Validate your client's feelings and experiences as much as you honestly can. Self-disclosure is often a good way to do this.

  I can see that you are very angy about Wally's lack of progress. I can tell that you care about him a lot and it must be frustrating to see him feeling so poorly. I am frustrated too and want what is best for him. Would you be willing to meet with me so that we can discuss your concerns more thoroughly?
- Use open-ended questions to understand your client's needs, problems, complaints, and concerns:

  I can tell that you love Wally a lot. I want what is best for him, too. What is it that you need today?
- Communicate empathy and apologize if appropriate:

  I can see that you are very angry about the delay. I'm sorry that you had to wait. Can we talk for a few minutes about Snowball's surgery?
- Set limits regarding your client's behavior and the kind of communication you will not tolerate:

  I want to help you with Wally and want to hear your concerns, but I can't help you while you are yelling at me.

  I'd like to help but I won't if you continue to put me down.
- Use gentle confrontation and paraphrasing to help your client explore deeper feelings underneath the anger:

  I understand you are very angry about Barney's death. I also get the sense that your feelings of sadness run very deep and are causing you great pain. It's sad to lose such a wonderful friend. Sometimes anger is a part of grief. I wonder if you're really angry with me or if you're just plain angry at the fact that Barney died.
- Sometimes, despite your best efforts, you cannot diffuse a client's anger by yourself. If you're unable to calm the client, refer to a colleague for assistance.

It is also important to develop and maintain good self-care skills when confronted with angry clients. Remember that you are not responsible for the way in which clients express their anger, and you can only do your best in responding to them with openness and sincerity. Being around angry people can be very draining. Remind yourself that there is more to your life than just your work and take the extra time to participate in activities and hobbies that you enjoy outside work.

Some people use anger as a mask for other emotions they are feeling as a result of a pet's illness or death

How Will I Know if I've Been Successful?

When you've successfully managed another person's anger, you can usually uncover the cause of it and address the person's needs. When clients are able to tell you what they need or want, you can then employ all your other helping strategies to work through the issue.

Remember that as a care provider, you are in a position of power because the pet owner needs or wants something from you (a healthier pet, reassurance, understanding). If clients realize that being angry or yelling at you will not help them to get what they want, the anger will usually lessen.

Strategies:

____

____

____

____

____

____

____

____

____

____

____

____

Situation 14

Clients with Financial Constraints

Jennifer arrives at your clinic with her six-month-old Siberian Husky puppy named Juno. Juno has been sick for two days. Jennifer is visibly worried and anxious. She tells you that she got Juno right after breaking up with her boyfriend of six years and that Juno has gotten her through the pain and sorrow of the last few months. Your diagnostic tests reveal that Juno has a parvovirus infection and that the prognosis is fairly good, but only if you can pursue aggressive treatment right away. Treatment will require at least two to three days of hospitalization. You give Jennifer a price estimate for the treatment and she begins to cry, telling you that she can't possibly afford this treatment. She tells you that her ex-boyfriend took her car and neglected to pay many bills from the apartment that they were sharing together. She says that she's badly in debt and appeals to you to "help save her baby."

What's Going on Here?

Discussing money and the cost of veterinary services presents a challenge to most veterinarians. The issue of money is particularly difficult because it almost always involves high levels of emotion as well as frequent life and death situations for the animal. *Financial issues are almost inevitably paired with the perception of care and compassion.* This is unfortunate because no one can put a price tag on compassion.

The difficult set-up for veterinarians is that many people measure your level of compassion in a monetary way. In addition, many pet owners have very unrealistic ideas and expectations about the cost of veterinary services. The average pet owner does not appreciate and understand all that is involved in quality veterinary care. In fact, some pet owners do not even know how much education, time, and training you have invested in becoming a veterinarian.

The difficult set-up for veterinarians is that many people measure your level of compassion in a monetary way.

Many pet owners think of veterinary care in the same financial terms as they do their own medical care; care that is usually covered by insurance companies. As a result, many people have little appreciation for the true costs of human medical services. For example, they might make a $10.00–$20.00 co-payment or pay 20 percent for a surgery that actually costs thousands of dollars. Since insurance is extremely rare in veterinary medicine, pet owners pay the full price of services without really understanding how inexpensive veterinary medical care is compared to human medical care. It's hard for a person to understand why a radiograph for their cat costs $50.00 when the radiograph of their own foot cost them only $20.00.

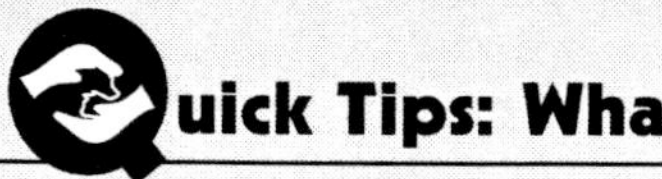

Quick Tips: What to Say, What to Do

- Set limits ahead of time. Make your payment policy clear at the very beginning of the appointment to avoid misunderstandings later on.
- Validate and acknowledge your client's reaction to financial limitations. Be aware that the client may be feeling scared, shocked, embarrassed, angry, or guilty about not being able to afford veterinary services. Whenever possible, try to preserve the client's self-esteem:

  It must be frightening to realize how much effort it is going to take to treat Juno. I know that her illness is a real shock to you.

  I can see that you are surprised by the cost of this surgery and really want to help Juno. You obviously care for her very much and were not expecting this sudden expense.
- De-personalize your clients' comments if they get angry. When clients vent their frustration, it is usually more about them than it is about you. Some clients can become desperate and may appeal to your sense of guilt by asking, "Don't you care about animals?" In these situations, it is helpful to make the client understand that your financial limitation does not reflect your level of compassion any more than it does for them:

  Jennifer, I know how much you love Juno. I care about her, too. However, just as your financial constraints do not reflect how much you love her, my commitment to her cannot be judged by my own financial limitations. I'd like to see if we can work together and find some options that will allow us both to help Juno the best way that we can, given both of our financial needs.
- Use self-disclosure to let clients know that you do understand and care:

  Finances are one of the toughest parts of my job. I do this work because I love animals and I feel sad and frustrated when I can't help them for free.
- Educate clients about your costs. Demonstrate the procedures you performed:

  It sounds like you have some concerns about your bill. We're dedicated to providing quality health care for Juno and that caliber of care quickly adds up. Would you like me to show you some of what we did and talk about the services we provided for her today?
- Provide written information and estimates for the medical procedures you perform and prepare the client for possible future expenses. Have clients sign the estimates and provide a range for the potential costs involved with a particular medical procedure. Allow for a cushion when you give a price range but don't over-estimate too much so as to "scare" the client away.
- Explore other options. Try to keep the client the responsible party for figuring out how to pay for the animal's treatment. Alternatives might include finding family or friends who will lend your client a credit card, getting an advance on a paycheck, or even borrowing the money from a friend or a bank (instead of from you!).

Another factor is a simple lack of education or planning. Some people buy or adopt animals impulsively without thinking through all the financial consequences. Still others have little understanding about the medical needs of their animals and find themselves unprepared when problems arise.

Your most valuable tool in talking about money is client education. If you can find the extra fifteen minutes, you can often answer your client's money-based questions and explain the cost of their animal's care. When discussing money, it is important for you to expect that your client may have high emotions and for you to be adequately prepared to deal with those emotions.

How Can I Connect?

First and foremost, you should determine ahead of time if money issues will be a personal hook for you. For many veterinarians it is, while for others, it isn't. If you know ahead of time how you might potentially react to these situations, you will be adequately prepared to deal with them when they arise. *The key is to uncouple your sense of compassion from your responsibility to your business and providing good medical care.*

You cannot possibly provide quality medical care if you are constantly undercharging for your services. Remind yourself that having a commitment to your business, employer, or your family's financial well-being does not mean that you do not love animals. You, and possibly your employer, will determine if and when there are special circumstances under which you might discount or provide complimentary veterinary services.

Other strategies you might use are to:

- donate a small percentage of profits to create a client subsidy fund. Some veterinary practices create special funds for unusual circumstances like animal abuse or emergencies. Employees can donate to these funds as well as clients who might want to memorialize an animal in a special way. Clients like the idea of helping other animals and owners who are in financial need.
- promote pet health insurance.
- be consistent, both personally and in your practice. When you do reduce a fee or give away your services, be aware that there may be consequences. People talk and share information. You might feel terrific after financially helping Mrs. Brown save her little beagle, but you may have more problems that you expected when the ladies in Mrs. Brown's church group do not understand why you can't do the same for their pets.

Remember to believe in the value of your services. You have worked very hard and put forth a substantial financial investment to obtain your degree and level of training. You provide a valuable service and deserve to be compensated for those services. Remembering this will help you to separate your sense of compassion from your financial responsibilities and help you to deal with emotional conversations involving money.

How Will I Know if I've Been Successful?

There will likely be many financial situations in your practice that will frustrate you, challenge you, and tug at your heart strings. You might end up euthanizing when you would really prefer to treat, or end up watching a client leave your office upset and frustrated. You have limits and cannot help every unfortunate animal or owner. The best that you can do is communicate openly, provide as much education as possible, and act creatively to meet your patient's and client's needs. When you have made a sincere effort to help a client and animal without taking on their responsibility as a pet owner, you have acted in a compassionate, professional manner.

Strategies:

Situation 15

Grieving Clients

Client:	*I'm so sorry I'm crying. I shouldn't be crying...*
Veterinarian:	*It's okay to cry, Mary. I'd cry, too, if I learned that my dog had cancer.*

What's Going on Here?

Crying is one of the classic non-verbal signs of grief. People cry when they are grieving because it is a natural reaction to emotional pain. Crying is an effective way to release emotion and an essential part of the grieving process. Still, like the client in the opening dialogue, many people feel embarrassed or ashamed of their emotional outbursts.

One of the biggest obstacles to connecting with grieving clients is probably your own fear that you may cry, too. It's not uncommon for veterinarians to abruptly end conversations with clients because they are afraid that they themselves might "lose control" in a professional situation.

How Can I Connect?

People generally feel better after crying. In one study, researchers found that widows who had friends who encouraged them to cry were healthier than widows who experienced less encouragement from others to cry and to discuss their feelings of grief. It follows, then, that the best way to connect with your grieving clients is to encourage them to "get it out." Allow them to sob, wail, sniffle, and talk. If clients exhibit extreme displays of emotion, like panic attacks or sobbing, help them work through their waves of emotion. Never leave the room because you assume your clients want to be alone. The act of leaving the room may signal your own embarrassment or disapproval of their grief. All forms of grieving (with the exception of responses that may be physically harmful to the client or to someone else) are healthy and acceptable forms of communication. Your job as a skilled communicator is to become comfortable with grief.

You can learn more about connecting with grieving clients in *The Practical Guide to Grief*, Book One of AAHA's "Building the Client Bond" series.

> Your job as a skilled communicator is to become comfortable with grief.

How Will I Know if I've Been Successful?

Most veterinarians also grieve when their patients die and it is important for you to remember that your emotional responses to loss are normal, too. Most clients feel comforted by their veterinarian's tears, but, whether you cry or not, you may find it helpful to express your feelings or to take a few minutes for yourself to grieve in your own way. You will know you are dealing with patient death successfully when, instead of hardening yourself to the emotional ramifications of death, you allow yourself to actually feel the emotions that accompany loss and find ways to grieve.

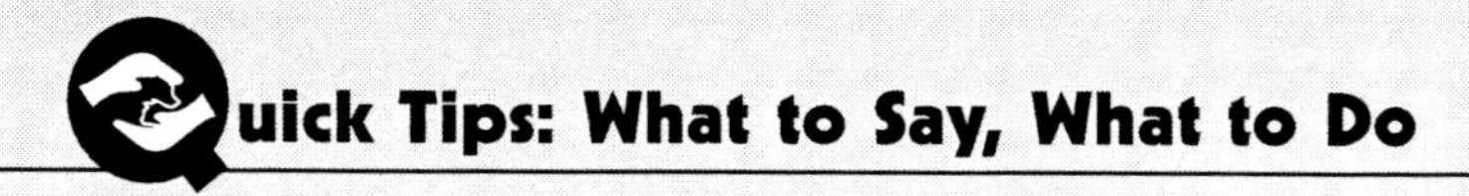

Quick Tips: What to Say, What to Do

- Acknowledge your client's grief:
  I can see how sad you are about Freddie's diagnosis.
- Normalize your client's tears:
  I would expect you to cry in a situation like this.
- Give permission to cry. Offer your client a tissue, a place to sit down:
  Take your time and let it out, Mary. I'm right here for you.
- Touch if providing non-verbal comfort is appropriate.
- Self-disclose by crying yourself if you're moved to do so. Crying demonstrates compassion and shows empathy for pets and their owners. If you cry easily you might say:
  I often cry during times like this. I can still do my job, though, and be here for you.
- If you cry easily, you might also try switching your focus from what you are feeling to what you are thinking. In studies where researchers have asked people what they are crying about, people usually stop crying in order to think of an answer.

Strategies:

The Telephone and Client Relations

The telephone can be a powerful client relations tool when it is used by a skilled communicator. Remember, when you use the telephone, your voice is your most powerful tool. Pay special attention to your voice tone, the pitch of your voice, and the pacing of your words:

- prepare yourself for potentially emotional calls by finding a quiet, controlled environment where you won't be distracted or interrupted.
- if you don't reach your client, do not leave details about emotional topics like a pet's death, relapse, or body care arrangements on voice mail or answering machines. Just leave a message, asking your client to return your call.
- maintain your client's confidentiality. If another family member or a co-worker answers or even returns your call, don't give them the details about your patient's condition. Simply leave the same message, asking your client to return your call or call back yourself at another time.
- if a client has not returned your call within a reasonable amount of time, call again. Messages get lost and clients, especially emotional ones, sometimes forget to return calls. It's your responsibility to make contact with your client and you must keep trying until that task is accomplished.
- when you call a client at work, he or she may be unable to talk freely with you about emotional issues at that time as they may not have any privacy. Before you begin, tell them you need to discuss a difficult issue with them and ask them if this is a convenient time to talk or if they would prefer to arrange a telephone appointment when they can speak more freely from a private area.
- give clients choices regarding how much detail and the kind of information you share with them. For example, you might say, "I would be happy to explain the details of Misty's surgery to you. Would you like that information now?" Each client's need for details varies, so it's best to ask rather than overwhelm your client with information.

Caught in the Act

I Appreciate what You Did!

Name ______________________________ Date ______________

Your Excellent Example of Effective Communication was:

(To be filled out by colleagues who observe *or* clients who experience outstanding communication exchanges.)

Thanks for being clear and honest!
Signed,

____

Communication Feedback Form

Three Praises and a Wish

On a scale of 1 to 5, with 5 being outstanding, rate your own or your colleague's performance in each area appropriate to an act of client communication. Include specific ideas regarding what you or your colleague did well and what needs to be improved. Discuss results at staff meetings.

Client Communication Techniques

Performance Area	Rating (1=poor, 5=outstanding)	Performance Area	Rating (1=poor, 5=outstanding)
Acknowledging	________	Structuring the Environment	________
Normalizing	________	Attending	________
Giving Permission	________	Active Listening	________
Asking Tough Questions	________	Use of Silence	________
Paraphrasing	________	Minimal Encouragers	________
Self-Disclosing	________	Responding with Touch	________
Gentle Confrontation	________	Written Materials	________
Immediacy	________	Demonstrations	________

Three Praises

You performed especially well in these three areas. I was impressed!

____

____

A Wish

You could improve in this area. Keep practicing!

____

____

References

1. McKey, E. and K. Payne. "APPMA study: pet ownership soars." *Pet Business* Vol. 18 (8): 22–23, 1992.

2. Voith, V. L. "Attachment of people to companion animals." In Quackenbush, J., and Voith, V. L., eds. *Veterinary Clinics of North America (Small Animal Practice)*, 15: 289–296, 1985.

3. The 1995 AAHA Report: A Study of the Companion Animal Veterinary Services Market. AAHA, Lakewood, CO, 1995.

4. American Pet Products Manufacturers Association. "Survey of pet owner ship in the USA." *Pet Business*, Vol. 14 (8), August, 1988.

5. Friedmann, E., Katcher A. H., Lynch, J. J. and Thomas, S. A. "Animal companions and one-year survival of patients after discharge from a coronary care unit." *California Veterinarian*. 8: 45–50, 1982.

6. Friedmann, E., Katcher, A. H., Lynch, J. J. and Thomas, S. A. "Animal companions and one-year survival of patients after discharge from a coronary care unit." *Pub. Health Report* 95 (4): 307–312, 1980.

7. Antelyes, J. "Client hopes client expectations." *JAVMA* 197 (12): 1596–1597, 1990.

8. Peters, R. 1987. *Practical Intelligence*. Harper and Row, NY. p. 96.

9. Troutman, C. M. *The Veterinary Services Market for Companion Animals*. Overland Park, Kansas, Charles, Charles Research Group and the American Veterinary Medical Association, Schaumburg, Il, 1988.

10. Soares, C., Mader, B. and B. Carmack. "Effective responses to the stress of pet death." Abstract in the *Proceedings of the Delta Society Annual Conference*, Parsippany NJ, 1989, p. 2.

11. Anonymous. "Communicate to avoid malpractice claims." *AVMA Trust Report* 10 (3): 1–2, 1991.

12. Steil, L. K., Summerfield, J., and G. deMare. *Listening, it can change your life: A handbook for scientists and engineers*. McGraw Hill Book Company, New York, 1983.

13. Schramm, W. "How communication works" by Wilbur Schramm, ed., in *The process and effects of mass communication*. University of Illinois, Urbana, IL, 1954, pp. 3–4.

14. Berlo, D. K. "The process of communication: An introduction to theory and practice." Holt, New York, 1960.

15. Soares, C., Mader, B. and B. Carmack. "Effective responses to the stress of pet death." Abstract in the *Proceedings of the Delta Society Annual Conference*, Parsippany NJ, 1989, p. 2.

16. Antelyes, J. "On being compassionate." *JAVMA* 190 (12): 1534–1536, 1987.

17. Mehrabian, A. "Communication without words." *Psych. Today*, September, 1968, p. 53.

18. Thompson, D. (ed.) *The Pocket Oxford Dictionery of Current English, eighth edition*. Clarendon Press, Oxford, 1992.

19. Campbell, J.H. and H.W. Helper. "Persuasion and interpersonal relationships" by J.H. Campbell and H.W. Helper, eds., in *Dimensions in Communication: Readings, Second edition*. Wadsworth Publ. Co., Belmont, CA, 1970, pp. 132-137.

20. Satir, V. *The new people making*. Science and Behavior Books, Mountain View, CA., 1988.

Resources

Communication Techniques Training Programs

Changes: The Support for People and Pets Program
Colorado State University Veterinary Teaching Hospital
300 West Drake
Fort Collins, CO 80523
Tel: 970-491-1242

Changes can provide information, education, and training about the communication techniques discussed in this book.

Audio and Video Tapes about Communication

"Friends for Life: Loving and Losing Your Animal Companion"
Lagoni, L., Butler, C., and Hetts, S.
This tape set discusses typical examples of interspecies communication, as well as subjects like animal behavior and companion animal euthanasia.
Sounds True Audio
P.O. Box 8010
Boulder, CO 80306-8010
Tel: 1-800-333-9185
FAX: 303-665-5292

Books about Communication

There are hundreds of books on the market about communication. Many address specific situations like anger or specific communication styles like those attributed to gender differences. Some of the more well-known books are listed here. Check with your local library or book store for other books appropriate to your needs.

Arapakis, M. *Softpower! How to Speak Up, Set Limits, and Say No Without Losing Your Lover, Your Job, or Your Friends.* Warner Books, New York, 1990.

Bilodeau, L. *The Anger Workbook*, CompCare Publishers, Minneapolis, MN, 1992.

Bolton, R. *People Skills: How to Assert Yourself, Listen to Others, and Resolve Conflicts.* Simon & Schuster, New York, 1979.

Bramson, R. *Coping with Difficult People... in Business and in Life.* Ballantine Books, New York, 1981.

Foster, C. *There's Something I Have to Tell You: How to Communicate Difficult News in Tough Situations*. Harmony Books, New York, 1997.

Frey, W. *Crying: The Mystery of Tears*. Winston Press, Minneapolis, MN, 1985.

Gabor, D. *Speaking Your Mind in 101 Difficult Situations*. Simon & Schuster, New York, 1994.

Goleman, D. *Emotional Intelligence: Why it can matter more than IQ*. Bantam Books, New York, 1995.

Gray, J. *Men are from Mars, Women are from Venus*. HarperCollins Publishers, New York, 1992.

Lagoni, L., Butler, C., and Hetts, S. *The Human-Animal Bond and Grief*. W.B. Saunders Company, Philadelphia, PA, 1994.

Lundberg, G. and Lundberg, J. *I Don't Have to Make Everything All Better: A Practical Approach to Walking Emotionally with Those You Care About While Empowering Them to Solve Their Own Problems*. Riverpark Publishing Company, Las Vegas, NV, 1995.

McKay, M., Davis, M., and Fanning, P. *How to Communicate: The Ultimate Guide to Improving Your Personal and Professional Relationships*. MJF Books, New York, 1983.

McKay, M., Davis, M., and Fanning, P. *Messages: The Communication Skills Book*. New Harbinger Publications, Inc., Oakland, CA, 1995.

McKay, M., Fanning, P., Paleg, K., and Landis, D. *When Anger Hurts Your Kids: A Parent's Guide*. New Harbinger Publications, Inc., Oakland, CA, 1996.

Metcalf, C.W. and Felible, R. *Lighten Up: Survival Skills for People Under Pressure*. Addison-Wesley Publishing Company, Reading, MA, 1992.

Nirenberg, J. *Getting Through to People*. Prentice-Hall, Inc., Englewood Cliffs, NJ, 1963.

Satir, V. *The New Peoplemaking*. Science and Behavior Books, Inc, Mountain View, CA, 1988.

Smith, M. *When I Say No, I Feel Guilty*. Bantam Books, New York, 1975.

Steil, L., Summerfield, J., and deMare, G. *Listening: It Can Change Your Life. A Handbook for Scientists and Engineers*. McGraw-Hill Book Company, New York, 1983.

Tannen, D. *That's Not What I Meant!* Ballantine Books, New York, 1986.

Tannen, D. *Talking from 9 to 5. Women and Men in the Workplace: Language, Sex, and Power*. Avon Books, New York, 1994.

Woititz, J. and Garner, A. *Lifeskills for Adult Children*. Health Communications, Inc, Deerfield Beach, FL, 1990.

Glossary

Acknowledging: to recognize the existence or truth of something.

Active Listening: to listen for feelings, rather than the factual content of conversations.

Attending: body language that lets the person who is talking know that careful attention is being paid to what is being said.

Body Language: communication through gestures, poses, postures, facial expressions, eye contact, and movements.

Communicate: to succeed in conveying information; to be connected.

Confidentiality: to keep secret or private any information that is entrusted to you about another's personal life.

Congruent: an agreement of fit.

Demonstrations: to show or explain by experience or practical use.

Gentle Confrontation: a question or a statement used to point out discrepancies or inconsistencies in what has been said or done or used to set limits on clients' behaviors or expectations.

Giving Permission: encouraging clients to think, feel, and behave however they need to (within safe limits) without fear of judgment.

Human-Animal Bond: a popular way of referring to the types of relationships and attachments people form with animals, particularly companion animals. Also, an accepted area of scholarly research.

Immediacy: commenting on what is occurring in the present moment.

Non-Verbal: not involving words or speech.

Normalizing: lending credibility to others' thoughts, feelings, behaviors, and experiences.

Rapport: a harmonious relationship or communication.

Role Play: acting out characters and/or situations as an aid to developing empathy for others as well as improving specific skills and techniques.

Self-Disclosure: briefly sharing a personal experience when it may be appropriate and of use to someone else.

Structuring the Environment: adapting the physical elements of an environment to better meet the situation at hand.

Technique: the skillful use of a tool.

Touch: providing comfort and demonstrating care and concern by use of physical contact.

Trust: a firm belief in the reliability, truth or strength of someone or something.

Verbal: oral, not written.

Meet the Authors

Laurel Lagoni

Laurel Lagoni earned a Master's degree in Human Development and Family Studies from Colorado State University in 1984. In 1985, she co-founded Changes: The Support for People and Pets Program at the Colorado State University Veterinary Teaching Hospital (CSU-VTH) and co-directed the program until 1995. The Changes Program provides pet owners with grief education and support during emergencies, diagnoses, treatment procedures, decision-making, unexpected deaths, euthanasias, and bereavement follow-up. As a veterinary grief counselor with The Changes Program, Ms. Lagoni worked alongside veterinarians and veterinary technicians as a member of the case management teams and facilitated the emotional aspects of the CSU-VTH's medical cases.

As an instructor in the professional veterinary medical curriculum, Ms. Lagoni developed a comprehensive curriculum and taught thousands of students and veterinarians about the human-animal bond, effective communication and client relations techniques, veterinary grief counseling, and client-present euthanasia. She also co-authored the textbook entitled *The Human-Animal Bond and Grief* with Carolyn Butler, M.S. and Suzanne Hetts, Ph.D. (W.B. Saunders Company, 1994), and was a consultant to AAHA during the development of their Pet Loss videotape training series. Currently, Ms. Lagoni is the Managing Director of The Argus Center at Colorado State University.

Dana Durrance

Dana Durrance holds a Master's degree in Clinical Psychology from the University of Colorado at Denver. She is Assistant Director of Changes: The Support for People and Pets Program at the Colorado State University Veterinary Teaching Hospital. Ms. Durrance provides counseling, support, and education to pet owners during the diagnosis, treatment, or death of their companion animals. She assists owners with decision-making, and provides bereavement counseling and follow-up to individuals, children, and families, who come to the teaching hospital. She also provides support to clients during euthanasias.

Ms. Durrance teaches client-relations courses in the professional veterinary medical curriculum and helps students learn effective communication techniques and ways to support clients during times of grief and loss. She also teaches students protocols for helping during client-present euthanasia. In addition, she provides support to the hospital faculty, staff, and students as they relate to their own feelings around animal illness and death.

Ms. Durrance lives in Colorado Springs, Colorado with her husband (a practicing veterinarian), daughter, and two dogs.